FIRST PLACE BIBLE STUDY

$\mathcal{P}athway$ to
SUCCESS

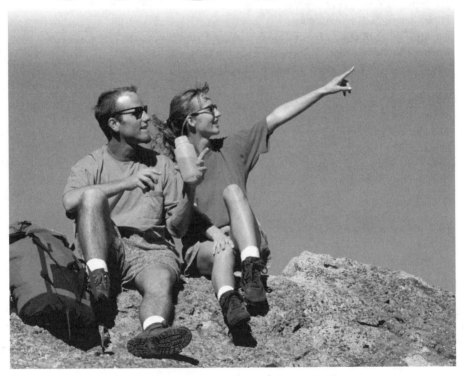

Gospel Light

FIRST PLACE™

PUBLISHING STAFF
William T. Greig, Chairman
Kyle Duncan, Publisher
Dr. Elmer L. Towns, Senior Consulting Publisher
Pam Weston, Senior Editor
Patti Pennington Virtue, Associate Editor
Jeff Kempton, Editorial Assistant
Hilary Young, Editorial Assistant
Bayard Taylor, M.Div., Senior Editor, Biblical and Theological Issues
Barbara LeVan Fisher, Packaging Concept and Design
Samantha A. Hsu, Cover and Internal Designer

CAUTION
The information contained in this book is intended to be solely informational and educational. It is assumed that the First Place participant will consult a medical or health professional before beginning this or any other weight-loss or physical-fitness program.

CONTENTS

FOREWORD

My introduction to Bible study came when I joined First Place in March of 1981. I had been in church since I was a small child, but the extent of my study of the Bible had been reading my Sunday School quarterly on Saturday night. On Sunday morning, I would listen to my Sunday School teacher as she taught God's Word to me. During the worship service, I would listen to our pastor as he taught God's Word to me. Digging out the truths of the Bible for myself had frankly never entered my mind.

Perhaps you are right where I was back in 1981. If so, you are in for a blessing you never dreamed possible. As you start studying the truths of the Bible for yourself, you will see God begin to open your understanding of His Word. Bible study is one of the nine commitments of the First Place program. The First Place Bible studies are designed to be done on a daily basis. Each day's study will take approximately 15 to 20 minutes to complete, but you will be discovering the deep truths of God's Word as you work through each week's study.

There are many in-depth Bible studies on the market. The First Place Bible studies are not designed for the purpose of in-depth study. They are designed to be used in conjunction with the other eight commitments of the program to bring balance into our lives. Our desire is for each member to begin having a personal quiet time with God each day. This time alone with God should include a time of prayer, Bible reading and Bible study. Having a quiet time is a daily discipline that will bring the rich rewards of balance, something we all need.

A part of each week's study is the Bible memory verse for the week. You will find a CD at the back of this Bible study that contains all 10 of the memory verses for the study set to music. The CD has an upbeat tempo suitable for use when exercising. The songs help you to easily memorize the verses and retain them for future reference. If you memorize Scripture as you study, God will use His Word to transform your life.

Almost every First Place member I have talked with about the program says, "The weight loss is wonderful, but the most important thing I have received from my association with First Place is learning to study God's Word."

God bless you as you begin this exciting journey toward a balanced life. God will richly bless your efforts to give Him first place in your life. Remember Matthew 6:33: "But seek first his kingdom and his righteousness, and all these things will be given to you as well."

Carole Lewis
First Place National Director

INTRODUCTION

The First Place Bible studies were developed to be used in conjunction with the First Place weight-loss program. However, the studies could also be used by anyone who desires to learn more about God's Word and His will, with the added bonus of learning more about living a healthy lifestyle.

A Balanced Life

First Place is a Christ-centered health program, emphasizing balance in the physical, mental, emotional and spiritual areas of life. The First Place program is meant to be a daily process. As we learn to keep Christ first in our lives, we will find that He is the One who satisfies our hunger and our every need.

God's Word contains guidelines for maintaining our physical well-being, equipping us mentally to make right choices, providing emotional stability to handle everyday circumstances as well as crisis situation, and growing spiritually as we deepen our relationship with Him.

The Nine Commitments

The First Place program has nine commitments that will help you draw closer to the Lord and aid you in establishing a solid, consistent and healthy Christian life. Each commitment is a necessary and important part of the goal of First Place: to help you become healthier and stronger in all areas of your life and live the abundant life He has planned for you. To help you achieve growth in all four areas, First Place asks you to keep these nine commitments:

1. Attendance
2. Encouragement
3. Prayer
4. Bible reading
5. Scripture memory verse
6. Bible study
7. Live-It plan
8. Commitment Record
9. Exercise

The Components

There are six distinct components to this Bible study to aid you in bringing balance to your life. These components include the 10-week Bible study, 6 Wellness Worksheets, 2 weeks of menu plans, the leader's discussion guide, 13 Commitment Records and the Scripture Memory Music CD.

The Bible Study

Each week of each 10-week Bible study is divided into five daily assignments with Days 6 and 7 set aside for reflections on the week's lesson. The following guidelines will help make your study more enjoyable and profitable:

- Set aside 15 to 20 minutes each day to complete the daily assignment. It's best not to attempt to complete a week's worth of Bible study in one day.
- Pray before each day's study and ask God to give you understanding and a teachable heart.
- Keep in mind that the ultimate goal of Bible study is not for knowledge only but also for application and a changed life.
- First Place suggests using the *New International Version* of the Bible to complete the studies.
- Don't feel anxious if you can't seem to find the *correct* answer. Many times the Word will speak differently to different people, depending upon where they are in their walk with God and the season of life they are experiencing.
- Be prepared to discuss with your fellow First Place members what you learned that week through your study.

Wellness Worksheets

The informative and interactive Wellness Worksheets have been developed by Dr. Jody Wilkinson of the Cooper Institute in Dallas, Texas. These worksheets are intended to help you understand and achieve balance in all four areas of your life: physical, mental, emotional and spiritual. Your leader will assign specific worksheets as At-Home Assignments throughout the 13-week session.

Menu Plans

The two-week menu plans were developed especially for First Place by Chef Scott Wilson. Each menu is meant to simplify meal planning and include food exchanges. These meals are based on the MasterCook software that uses a database of over 6,000 food items, which was prepared using United States Department of Agriculture (USDA) publications and information from food manufacturers.

Leader's Discussion Guide

This discussion guide is provided to help the First Place leader guide a group through this Bible study. It provides information for the leader to prepare for each weekly group meeting.

Personal Weight Record

The Personal Weight Record is for the member to use to keep a record of weight loss. After the weigh-in at each week's meeting, the member will record any loss or gain on the chart.

Commitment Records

Thirteen Commitment Records (CRs) are provided in the back of this Bible study. For your convenience these have been printed on perforated paper so that you may easily remove them from the book and carry them with you through each week as you keep your First Place commitments. Directions for filling out the CRs precedes those pages.

Scripture Memory Music CD

Since Scripture memory music is such a vital part of the First Place program, the Scripture Memory Music CD for this study is included in the back inside cover. The verses for this study are set to music that can be listened to as you work, play or travel. The CD can be an effective tool as you exercise since the first verse is set to music with a warm-up tempo, the next eight verses are set to workout tempo, and the music of the last verse can be used for a cooldown.

DREAM OF SUCCESS

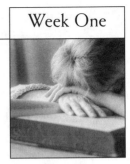

MEMORY VERSE
Where there is no revelation,
the people cast off restraint.
Proverbs 29:18

While browsing in a gift shop, Cindy noticed a beautifully framed piece of calligraphy. The words on the parchment read "Success is the progressive realization of a worthwhile dream." These simple yet profound words provoked a question in Cindy's heart: *What are the progressive steps along the path to success?* Over the next 10 weeks, together with the Lord, you and your First Place group will follow the path to success. The first step is to discover God's dream for you.

DAY 1: *Discover God's Dream for You*

An alternate translation of Proverbs 29:18 says "Where there is no vision, the people perish" *(KJV)*. God has a purpose for each of us. We know that everything He desires for us is good. God desires for us to be healthy and take care of our bodies. Proper nutrition and exercising are ways of implementing a vision, a dream, of what you will be as a result of following God's plan for you.

For Cindy, discovering God's dream for her life was not an easy task. After becoming a Christian at age 27 and joining First Place a couple of years later, Cindy began to catch a vision of what she could become with God's help. She dreamed of becoming a godly woman, wife and mother; of losing weight; of going to college; of leading a Bible study. Still, tough questions plagued Cindy. Could she really succeed? Could she change? Could she hope against hope? What about you and your hopes and dreams?

According to Jeremiah 33:3, God asks us to do something and promises to respond.

≫ What are we to do?

≫ What does God promise to do?

≫ In Psalm 37:5-6, what does God ask us to do?

≫ What is the result of following the instructions outlined in verse 6?

☐ God promises fulfillment

☐ God promises righteousness and justice as you commit to and trust Him.

≫ What is one of your dreams?

Perhaps you are without a dream, and you feel as though you are perishing. In this week's memory verse, Proverbs 29:18, the writer declared that people without revelation, a word from God, "cast off restraint." In other words, they live undisciplined lives. The disciplines of First Place help us lead a controlled life. Ask God to give you a dream, and resolve to lead a disciplined life that reflects your commitment to living obediently. Dreams give us purpose and direction. Living with appropriate restraint and discipline will help us attain our dreams.

➤ Have you ever thought, *I could accomplish so many wonderful dreams if I only had enough money?*

Reflect on the infinite riches God has given you in Christ Jesus, and then you can really begin to dream! His resources cannot be exhausted. He has a vision for your life. Rejoice today, for you have reason to hope. Believe that God will reveal Himself to you. His promises are as true today as they were centuries ago.

In your prayer journal today, ask God to show you the dream He has for your life. Ask Him to help you learn the memory verse—listen to the Scripture Memory Music CD and use *Walking in the Word* to help you learn the verse.

DAY 2: *Define Success*

Success has been defined as a favorable outcome. Thus, success is the achievement or completion of something. Is success merely completing a goal? Or do we find success along the way? Each step on the pathway toward the ultimate goal or dream is a step that spells success. Each step propels us to the next. Success breeds success! You have begun the journey! Today we will discover a biblical definition for success.

➤ Think of someone you view as successful. What do you think makes him or her successful?

In Joshua 1:1-9 God instructed Joshua about prosperity and success.

➤ Based on Joshua 1:1-9, list the words or phrases that describe conditions for success.

Obeying God's Word and seeking His will are key elements in defining God's concept of success. Verse 7 links success to obedience. Success in First Place and all other aspects of life, depends on our willingness to give Christ control in our lives.

≫ After rereading Joshua 1:8, summarize how God defines success.

A person who is seen as a failure in the world's view may be the most successful person in God's view.

 Father, I know You desire for me to be prosperous and successful. Holy Spirit, show me what success for me really is and how to find it. Help me to celebrate the joy of walking the path with You! I trust You to guide my footsteps.

DAY 3: *Surrender Shattered Dreams, Dare to Dream Again*

When Cindy was four years old, her parents divorced. Her father remarried and divorced again. Cindy entered adulthood and marriage with one driving conviction, one powerful dream. As long as it was in her power to control and prevent it, she would never allow divorce to happen to her or any future children. When divorce ended her 12-year marriage to her high school sweetheart, Cindy's heart broke. Would she ever dream again?

Have you had a dream that did not come true? Maybe you dreamed of being a more committed Christian or even shedding extra pounds. Perhaps you have experienced financial disaster, lost your job or been forsaken by friends or family. Have you felt like a failure because of disappointments with your children? If you have shattered dreams, you are not alone. Don't despair, there is hope.

Scripture records the lives of many people whose dreams and hopes were shattered.

❧ According to Genesis 29:16-30, what dream of Jacob's was shattered?

❧ How was Jacob's dream restored?

❧ Do you have any shattered dreams? If so, describe them here and/or in your prayer journal.

Have you surrendered these shattered dreams to God? If not, ask God to help you do so. Forgive anyone who may have hurt you, including yourself. You may even be angry at God. If so, tell Him how you feel.

Cindy endured the heartbreak of shattered dreams, but she made a decision to surrender those dreams to God. As she walked through the pain of divorce, Cindy found great strength to persevere in the lyrics of a simple chorus that reminded her that since Christ is alive, she could face the future. The message of this chorus inspired Cindy to dream of becoming a more devoted and committed Christian woman with God's help. She wanted God to shine through the cracks of the shattered life that He had put back together. You can dare to dream again too.

❧ According to Luke 23:44-49, what had shattered the disciples' dreams? What had happened to Jesus?

Consider the circumstances of the disciples when Jesus was arrested, beaten and crucified on the cross. The disciples' hopes and dreams were shattered. They faced life without a sense of purpose, hope or vision. They felt lost, aimless, hopeless, fearful and powerless until word came to them that Jesus was alive!

As you read John 20:17-29, put yourself in the disciples' place. How would you react? Being with Jesus restored the joy and faith of the disciples and relieved the doubts of Thomas.

➤ How does spending time with Jesus in prayer restore your faith in God's power?

➤ How does spending time with Jesus in prayer restore your faith in yourself?

Jesus restored the disciples' hope. Later He sent the Holy Spirit to comfort, guide and empower their lives. He gave the disciples a mission— a Kingdom purpose for which to live and die. Jesus can and will do the same for you.

➤ Are you afraid to dream again, afraid of being hurt or disappointed?

As you risk daring to dream again, consider the truths of these life-changing actions:

- 🍏 *Remember: Jesus is alive!* Because He lives you can face the past, the present and the future.
- 🍏 *Look to Jesus.* When you see Him, you will find grace, acceptance, strength and peace.
- 🍏 *Listen for His voice.* When you hear Him speak to your heart, His voice will give you reassurance, guidance and hope.
- 🍏 *Rely on His Word.* When you depend upon His Word, you will begin to know the purpose and mission God has planned for your life.
- 🍏 *Apply His power.* When you engage the power of the Holy Spirit, you can start over; you can dare to dream again!

Father God, I am willing to trust You with my new dreams, even my formerly shattered dreams. Please heal any wounds I have suffered from the loss of a dream. Give me new hope and boldness to dream anew.

DAY 4: *Evaluate Your Motives, Seek the Heart of God*

Most of her life Cindy struggled with being overweight. Beginning at an early age, she had been urged by her family to lose weight; as an adult, her husband encouraged it—even her insurance company had recently approached her about it. Nevertheless, nothing really motivated Cindy to lose weight, or at least not for very long. Finally, Cindy thought she had found the key she had been missing to unlock the gate of success. She simply wanted to lose weight for herself—to feel better, emotionally and physically! Did this new motivator work? Not for long. Eventually, Cindy learned that the most important motivation for losing weight is pleasing God.

Cindy discovered that God's love motivated her to want to please Him. Desiring to live a life that honors and glorifies her heavenly Father is the one driving force that holds her to His calling, keeps her on the right pathway and helps her persevere. When following the pathway toward a worthwhile dream, consider your motivation for pursuing it.

Examine your motivation for the dreams you have identified as a part of this week's study.

➣ Why do you want to be successful?

☐ To please myself
☐ To please someone else
☐ To please God

In the Sermon on the Mount (see Matthew 5:1-11), Jesus addressed the issue of right motives. In Matthew 6:1-18 Jesus addressed the issues of giving, praying and fasting.

≫ What is the common factor in each of these teachings?

≫ After reading Colossians 3:23-24, fill in the blanks to paraphrase Paul's teaching on motives.

Do whatever you do _____, as if you

were doing it for _____, not men.

≫ What is the reason we should do this?

≫ Think about why you joined First Place; is there someone other than God whom you are trying to please by focusing on healthy eating, fitness or losing weight?

☐ Yes   ☐ No

If your primary motive is to please, honor and obey God, then wanting to eat healthy, be physically fit or lose weight in order to feel better about yourself is not improper. Wanting your spouse, parents, family and friends to be proud of you is also legitimate. Most of us know that eating a balanced diet and leading a healthy lifestyle require more than our own willpower. It takes more than the encouragement of those who love us. Our willingness to let God have control of our lives will put us on the pathway to successful weight control.

King David was called a man after God's own heart (see Acts 13:22). Though David made many mistakes and committed many sins, he loved God. We can learn a great deal from David about seeking God's heart.

➣ Read the following verses; then summarize the actions and the results of seeking the heart of God:

• Psalm 9:10

• Psalm 37:4

• Psalm 40:8

• Psalm 63:1-5

• Psalm 86:11

➣ In what ways are you seeking the heart of God? Check all that apply.

☐ Personal Bible study time
☐ Scripture reading and memorization
☐ Daily prayer and quiet time
☐ Christian music, inspirational tapes
☐ Church attendance
☐ Christian conferences, retreats
☐ Christian radio
☐ Group Bible study classes/courses
☐ Others: _____

In the process of finding a worthwhile goal or dream, we must seek the heart of God. When we seek God, we will not desire those things that are contrary to His will. His desires will become ours, and He can reveal to us the vision He has for our lives.

As a youngster, spending time with her dad helped Cindy know the dreams he had for her life. Cindy knew the heart of her father so well that she seldom had to be told what displeased him. In fact, her conscience was deeply pierced when she disobeyed. Cindy desired to please her father even more as she grew to understand his love for her. Yet Cindy's earthly father was imperfect. He made mistakes in life and in parenting—and he even let Cindy down at times.

Our heavenly Father will never hurt us. He is a perfect Father. Just as each of us can know the heart of our earthly father, we can know the intent of God's heart. If we seek Him first through spending time with Him, He will give us those desires that originally come from His heart.

 Heavenly Father, give me a passion for serving You with an obedient, willing spirit. Help me have pure and righteous motives as I pursue Your dreams and goals for my life.

God, draw me closer to Your heart. You are my Father. Reveal the depth of Your love for me.

DAY 5: *Share Your Dream with Others*

Sharing our deepest longings, hopes and dreams may be easier for some than others, but God's Word supports the need for us to open our hearts. As we conclude this first week, consider the importance of sharing your dreams with others. Prepare to participate, if you are willing, during the Bible study time.

➤ According to Ruth 1:11-18 and 4:9-17, what dream of Naomi's was lost and then fulfilled?

➤ What dream of Ruth's was lost but then fulfilled?

First, Ruth had to be willing to share her dream with Naomi (see Ruth 2:19-23). Then, God used Naomi to help Ruth realize her dream (see Ruth 3:1-13).

➤ How can sharing your dreams with your First Place group members help you accomplish them?

➤ What are the potential advantages of sharing your dreams with others?

➤ What fears or hesitations could someone have about sharing their dreams?

Sharing your dreams with others will encourage you and may serve to encourage others. Ask the Lord to give you a heart that is willing to be vulnerable. Ask Him to provide friends whom you can trust—friends who will love you unconditionally as He does. Ask Him to give you friends who will pray for you, help you when you stumble and rejoice with you on the progressive pathway of success. Tell Him you are willing to be this kind of friend to someone else.

Listen closely as First Place members share their dreams, and ask God to touch your heart with the name of someone He wants you to support with a short e-mail, note of encouragement or a brief call. Lift that person up to the Lord in prayer today.

 Dear Lord, thank You that I can trust You with my hopes and dreams. Help me to be open to sharing them with others, and to be an encourager when others share their hopes and dreams with me. Walk with me in my vulnerability and guide me with Your unconditional love.

DAY 6: *Reflections*

If you have previously attended a First Place Bible study, you have hopefully discovered the power of learning to pray the Scriptures, which are a part of the optional reflection days of each weekly Bible study. Many of these wonderful Scripture prayers are from Beth Moore's book *Praying God's Word*.[1] If this is your first session of First Place, you will have the opportunity to learn how to use this powerful tool to change your prayer life.

As you prepare to meet with the group, give thanks to God that you are not alone on the path. Ask the Lord to help group members form a strong bond. Determine to grow closer to at least one other person in the group each week and to depend on Christ to help you each day. For example, begin the habit of writing your prayers each day; ask your leader for help to better understand the food plan; encourage someone in the group by sending a note; review your memory verse with a friend; thank the Lord for your leader; find a walking partner.

Faithful, loving Lord, according to Your Word, two are better than one, because they have a good return for their work: If one falls down, his friend can help him up. But pity the man who falls and has no one to help him up (see Ecclesiastes 4:12)! Please help me to form healthy relationships and find support in those who encourage me to get back on my feet and walk with You when I fall. Help me to remember that You and I and a good friend to hold me accountable are like a cord of three strands that is not easily broken.[2]

Father, as we begin this journey, help each of us in the group to depend on You and to support each other so we will be stronger. I praise You for the promise of the blessing of a good return for our work (see Ecclesiastes 4:9). I pray that each one of us who begins this session will commit to completing it.

Lord, You have assured me in Your Word that two are better than one, because they will receive a good benefit for all of their efforts. Therefore, I truly believe that You have brought our First Place group members together, because we will be able to be more successful as we help each other during this session. If one of us has a tough week, others can lend support and encouragement to get going again. How pitiful it would be to try to do this all alone. Father, thank You for the help You will bring to me through this group. Together, with Your mighty help, we can stand against any foe!

DAY 7: *Reflections*

The focus of this first week's study has been to learn the importance of dreams in relation to success. Don't be afraid to dream. Don't be afraid of difficulties.

Among your dreams and goals, have you included a vision of a more intimate relationship with Christ? Scripture memorization is one important pathway in developing this intimacy. God's Word is also your weapon against Satan in the struggles and temptations of everyday life (which will be discussed in more detail in week four). Psalm 119:11 says, "I have hidden your word in my heart that I might not sin against you." You are encouraged to begin this session of First Place with a compelling passion to know Christ more and a heartfelt commitment to hide God's Word in your heart.

If possible, spend a little time outdoors today, perhaps in a garden or park. God's presence in nature is unmistakable. Our Lord is the creator of the universe, yet He invites us to share an intimate, one-on-one relationship with Him. If we will listen carefully, we will hear Him speak to our hearts. Freely respond to His invitation. Offer Him your dreams; offer Him a heart and life filled with praise to the One who created you.

Review this week's memory verse, use the Scripture Memory Music CD and the *Walking in the Word* book often.

 "Sovereign LORD, you have made the heavens and the earth by your great power and outstretched arm. Nothing is too hard for you" (Jeremiah 32:17).

Lord, You said if we ask it will be given to us, if we seek we will find and if we knock the door will be opened to us. Lord, I ask You to take my dreams that fall in line with Your will for my life and show me how to realize each one. Help me to daily seek You and to follow the First Place commitments. Thank You for opening the door and showing me the path to take (see Luke 11:9).

Almighty God, You said that where there is no vision—no divine revelation—the people perish. Father, I need and want Your vision for my life. Give me Your revelation so that my life is directed and disciplined (see Proverbs 29:18, *KJV*).

Not by my might or power, Lord, but by Your Spirit, I will entrust my dreams to You and walk the pathway to success (see Zechariah 4:6).

Notes

1. Beth Moore, *Praying God's Word* (Nashville, TN: Broadman and Holman, 2000).
2. Ibid., pp. 163-164.

GROUP PRAYER REQUESTS   TODAY'S DATE:_____

NAME	REQUEST	RESULTS

PLAN FOR SUCCESS

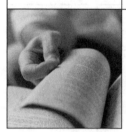

MEMORY VERSE
*May he give you the desire of your heart
and make all your plans succeed.*
Psalm 20:4

In her book *Free to Dream*, Neva Coyle states: "A healthy wish [dream] propels us into the future—the minutes, days, months, years ahead that are now beyond our sight."[1] With our dreams in mind, we now stand on the second stepping-stone of the pathway to success: plan for success. Just as every contractor needs a set of building plans before construction begins, the path to success requires a plan of action—a blueprint of sorts. In this week's study we will discover what God's Word has to say about His plan for successfully fulfilling our dreams.

DAY 1: *Trust God*

In last week's study we met a woman named Cindy who found in Jeremiah 29:11 not only God's assurances, but also strength and confidence to face the unknown.

➤ According to this verse, what kind of plans does God have for us?

    Facing life as a single parent with three young children, Cindy relied on God's promise of a hope and a future. Later, when her son fought in Operation Desert Storm during the Gulf War and when her daughter experienced a difficult and life-threatening childbirth, Cindy remembered again God's promise. She found comfort in knowing that His plans are to prosper—not to harm—His children.

➤ What gives you confidence to face the future? Do you rest in the faithful assurances of God's Word?

➤ How does your participation in First Place contribute to fulfilling God's promise found in Jeremiah 29:11?

➤ How does God want to prosper you?

When reading Jeremiah 29:11, perhaps you thought: *God may know His plans for me, but I haven't got a clue! I wish He would reveal His plans to me.* If so, you are not alone. Most Christians feel this way at one time or another. None of us knows the future. Faith may mean taking a step onto a new and unfamiliar path. If we always knew where each step would lead, the Christian life would not be called a faith walk. When you feel the dark clouds of life hiding God's plan for you, remember His promise in Jeremiah 29:11.

After reading Psalm 91, underline in your Bible the words that indicate where we find safety from life's storms or write them in the margin of your Bible.

➤ Write at least one word or phrase from the verses in Psalm 91 that gives you assurance in God, and explain why this is meaningful for you.

 Father, when I feel lost and without hope or a future, help me to run to You—to the only sure place where I will find safety. Help me to run to Your refuge, God. Then cradle me in Your bosom so that I will grow closer to the heart of You, the One who has wonderful plans for my life.

Lord, I want to be closer to You, for You love me beyond measure, and desire to prosper me and give me hope and a future.

DAY 2: *Count the Cost*

As a single mom, Cindy learned self-reliance. In fact, she became too self-reliant. She found herself making plans apart from God and then submitting them to Him for approval. She often wondered why God didn't bless her plans. She had to learn to seek God's plans first and then make her plans according to His.

How does Psalm 18:30-32 describe God's plan?

If we make our own plans, we are not as likely to succeed. Though we often think we know what should be done, our plans are imperfect. We can trust God's plan, because He knows the future and His way is perfect.

➤ Read 2 Chronicles 26:3-5 and complete the following:

Uzziah did what was _____in the sight of God.

➤ Under what condition would Uzziah continue to prosper?

Read the rest of 2 Chronicles 26 to find out what happened to Uzziah. Do you truly seek God's plans? Are you confident that His way is best for you, or do you depend on and trust your own plans? Do you trust in something or someone besides God? Ask God to search your heart as you contemplate these questions.

꙳ How is First Place helping you seek God's leadership in all that you do?

Take a moment to ask God to help you relinquish any of your plans that are not also His plans for your life. Review this week's memory verse.

As you seek to implement God's plans for your life and prepare for the successful realization of your dreams or goals, be willing to count the cost. Consider the impact of your plans on all areas of your life, including any sacrifices that you may need to make.

In Luke 14:26-33, Jesus instructed His disciples to count the cost before making the life-changing decision to follow Him.

꙳ How does Jesus summarize the cost of being a disciple? Check one.

☐ You will have to give up comfort.

☐ You will have to give up riches.

☐ You will have to give up everything.

꙳ To accomplish your dreams and goals in the First Place program, what sacrifices will you need to make? Check all of the areas that will involve sacrifice for you.

☐ Exercise   ☐ Commitment Record
☐ Spiritual disciplines   ☐ Eating habits
☐ Time   ☐ Finances

꙳ What other things might you have to sacrifice to meet your goals?

One important cost to consider is the cost of your time. Pray about how you spend your time. Does your time management benefit you and bring glory to God?

⇛ What changes might you need to make in the area of time management?

To pursue your First Place goals, what does discipline cost? Discipline is involved in menu planning, grocery shopping, choosing smaller helpings and making healthier choices when eating out. You may need to stop serving a family member's favorite dessert if it tempts you. You may have to learn to set boundaries with people who seem to want to sabotage your efforts, whether innocently or intentionally.

Some exercise choices may have a monetary cost involved, such as fees related to an aerobics class, health-club membership, purchase of home exercise equipment or purchase of appropriate clothing and footwear. Ask God to provide you with the resources and to help you make any necessary sacrifices.

Above all, you must count the cost of developing your relationship with Jesus Christ. This relationship must change and grow more than any other, if you really want success. Deepening your relationship to Jesus Christ is worth whatever it costs.

Father, help me to set my heart on things above so that other life choices fall into their proper place. I want godly thoughts and desires to take precedence over earthly pleasures, which are temporary and may lead me away from Your plans (see Colossians 3:1).

Lord, help me sustain my determination, on a daily basis, to be willing to sacrifice—whatever the cost—to fulfill Your plan for me.

DAY 3: *Set Goals*

Cindy was often amazed at the ambition and perseverance of one of her friends. When Cindy asked her how she stayed on course, she answered, "I know where I am going and what it takes to get there." She had long-range goals.

Setting long-range goals is crucial to a plan for success. When you identified your dreams of success in week one, you may have formed one or more long-range goals. One of Cindy's long-range goals was to lose 100 pounds. Do you have a long-range goal?

In Philippians 3:10-14, Paul wrote to the believers in Philippi about his goals.

≫ From Philippians 3:10-14, describe Paul's long-range goals in your own words.

≫ What did Paul say he was doing to achieve his goal?

≫ What did he say about the past?

Focusing on past failures and accomplishments can impede our progress in reaching our goals for the future. For example, you may have tried to lose weight in the past without success—at least without permanent success. Thinking about that experience may keep you from believing you can lose and keep the weight off in First Place.

≫ List any personal long-range goals you may have.

Do you know where you are going and what you want to do with your life? Do you know what it will take to get there? Keep your long-range goals clearly defined and foremost in your thoughts each day. Allow them to motivate you to live by a higher standard and without compromise.

Take a few moments to copy into your prayer journal the long-range goals you have listed here.

We serve a God of order. His ultimate plans and purposes are carried out by definite steps of progression. God's long-range plans for you are achieved by smaller short-range goals.

➤ According to Joshua 6:1-20, what was the ultimate goal of the Israelites?

➤ What were the short-range goals of Days 1 through 6?

➤ What was the short-range goal of Day 7?

➤ What was required of the people for the ultimate goal to be achieved?

Commit yourself to achieving your short-range goals. Keep a record in your prayer journal. Solicit the help of others who will hold you accountable. Plan to reward yourself as you accomplish each goal. If in the past you have rewarded yourself with food, use other, more beneficial rewards. They can be as simple as taking a soaking bath, relaxing with a good book or taking a weekend trip.

➤ Look back at one of your long-range goals. Then list at least one short-range goal you must achieve to accomplish your long-range goal. Challenge yourself to take the first step today.

In your prayer journal, list short-range goals that lead toward the long-range goals that you have identified. Be specific. If you don't know your target, you'll miss the mark every time.

Father God, make Your goals for my life very clear, and then help me to accomplish them.

Lord, show me what I need to do today, this week, this month and this year that will move me closer to my long-range goals. Grace me daily to be steadfast in pursuing Your will for my life.

DAY 4: *Set Priorities*

If we want to realize our dreams in this fast-paced world, time management is crucial. Keeping our priorities in mind will help us achieve success.

➤ Carefully read Ecclesiastes 3:1-8; Luke 12:15-21 and Ephesians 5:15-17. Based on these verses, answer the following questions:

What should be your priority in the use of your time?

What are your greatest challenges to using your time wisely and setting priorities for your life?

Cindy found she needed to make changes in how she spent her time. You, too, may need to sacrifice time spent watching TV, going to the movies or reading the newspaper to allow time for Bible study, Scripture reading, exercise and group meetings.

Perhaps you will need to change your usual sleeping habits to allow time in the morning or evening for prayer.

➤ Have you established a special time for

Scripture reading?	☐ Yes	☐ No
Exercise?	☐ Yes	☐ No
Meal planning?	☐ Yes	☐ No
Commitment Record keeping?	☐ Yes	☐ No
Encouragement commitment?	☐ Yes	☐ No
Daily Bible study lesson?	☐ Yes	☐ No
Daily prayer/quiet time?	☐ Yes	☐ No
Reviewing weekly memory verse?	☐ Yes	☐ No

➤ List other activities that will help you to accomplish other personal goals.

Commit your time to God as you begin each day. Ask Him to help you redeem the time. Mark your calendar with your weekly First Place group meetings and exercise times. Schedule time with your family and loved ones. Allow 10 to 15 minutes of planning time at the start of each day; this will ultimately save you time. Include Sunday School and worship services in your weekly events. Above all, treasure each precious day of life that He gives you.

 Heavenly Father, help me to plan the wise use of the time You have given me and to make the most of every opportunity. Lord, help me to store up the things that are rich in You.

DAY 5: *Stay Flexible*

Now you have a plan for success. But are you prepared to cope with the unexpected things that inevitably alter your plans? The unexpected may happen by God's design or may come from the enemy's plan to distract us. We need to be flexible with our plans and be willing to make adjustments based on His leading.

➳ According to Acts 16:16-34, what had Paul expected to do before a demon-possessed girl interrupted his plans?

➳ Do you think Paul's actions reflected a heart willing to stay flexible?

☐ Yes   ☐ No

➳ What happened as a result of this interruption in Paul's plan?

➳ How do you react when you have to make a change in your plans?

➳ What is your typical response if you have to miss a group meeting or make adjustments in what you eat? Do you tend to give up and quit at the slightest interruption of your plans?

God, I entrust my plans to You, the master planner and designer. Help me to stay flexible and to be willing to let You create a new plan for my day if You so desire.

Loving Father, I need Your counsel daily. Help me to listen to Your still, small voice so that I can walk in Your wisdom.

DAY 6: *Reflections*

During this week's study we have discovered several important factors about planning that influence our potential for success. Reflect on the worthwhile dreams and goals you hope to progressively realize during this session. If you still need help to define your goals, two acrostics may prove beneficial to you. Combining the elements of these two acrostics with the power of praying the Scriptures will enable you to prepare for victory when the enemy tries to thwart God's plans for your life.

The first acrostic is SMART. Planning and setting SMART goals will help you to be more successful in reaching them. Compare your goals to the descriptions of the SMART goals. If adjustments or revisions are needed, take a few minutes to modify and fine-tune your goals. If you need more help defining your goals, call on someone in the group or ask a close friend or family member; call upon the Lord and seek His help too. Record any revisions in your prayer journal. SMART goals are

Specific and individual

Manageable and measurable

Attainable and reasonable

Realistic and challenging

Tangible and utilize time management

Continue to review this week's memory verse, using your Scripture Memory Music CD and *Walking in the Word* book. Also review the memory verse from week one. Pray through the following Scripture prayers as you undertake the plans you and the Lord have made this week.

You know the plans You have for me, O Lord. You have declared that they are plans to prosper me and not to harm me, plans to give me a hope and a future (see Jeremiah 29:11).[2]

Lord, for too long I have given the devil a foothold (see Ephesians 4:27).[3] Please help me to stop offering him so many opportunities to bring defeat into my life. Your plan for me is victory.

Faithful Father, I am prayerfully committing my way to You; trusting also in You; knowing You will bring it to pass. Help me to do my part, Lord (see Psalm 37:5).

Glorious God, how I celebrate the fact that my eyes have never seen, my ears have never heard and my mind has never conceived what You have prepared for me and all others who truly love You. Help me also to understand that this awesome plan is revealed to me by Your Spirit (see 1 Corinthians 2:9-10).[4]

Lord, according to Your Word, if I wholeheartedly commit whatever I do to You, my plans will succeed. Lord, I realize that the essence of committing any plan to You is seeking Your plan. Let me never forget to commit everything I do to You. Show me the right path, Father (see Proverbs 16:3).

Lord, teach me to delight in You. Your Word says that You will give me the desires of my heart when I delight in You. I want to delight in You above any other desire of my heart (see Psalm 37:4). Thank You for loving me so much. Thank You for Your plans to use First Place in my life. Help me to make SMART goals that will assist me in successfully accomplishing these plans.

DAY 7: *Reflections*

As mentioned in Day 6, two acrostics can prove helpful as you plan for success in reaching your goals. Not only should your goals be SMART, as you learned yesterday, but they also need to be WISE.

Planning and setting WISE goals can be an essential factor in helping you accomplish your dreams. Compare your goals to the fundamental elements of WISE goals. If adjustments or revisions are needed, take a few minutes to modify and fine-tune your goals. Record these in your prayer journal. Then note two or three specific ways you could bring about each of these concepts. WISE goals involve

Written, well-defined objectives with godly wisdom and action

Inspiration and motivation from God and others

Support and encouragement from family and friends

Evaluation and review of commitments and circumstances

Seek God's wisdom and power as you plan for success, and He will faithfully assist you.

 Lord, Your Word warns that "he who trusts in himself is a fool, but he who walks in wisdom is kept safe" (Proverbs 28:26).[5] I have come to realize that I cannot trust in myself. My safety is in learning to trust in You. Please help me to do just that.

I confess to You that I am overwhelmed by the task ahead, but am thankful that You have authority over all things. Heaven is Your throne and Earth Your footstool; therefore, anything over my head is under Your feet (see Matthew 5:34-35).[6]

"Show me your ways, O LORD, teach me your paths; guide me in your truth and teach me, for you are God my Savior, and my hope is in you all day long. Remember, O LORD, your great mercy and love, for they are from of old. Remember not the sins of my youth and my rebellious ways; according to your love remember me, for you are good, O LORD" (Psalm 25:4-7).[7]

Father, I rejoice in Your promise to me, just like someone who finds great treasure (see Psalm 119:162, NKJV). Thank You, Lord, for the promise of a plan for my life and for Your help as I establish WISE goals to implement those plans. I am excited about the journey ahead. I am trusting in You. Help me to follow Your guidance.

Almighty God, Your Word tells me to trust in You with all my heart and to not lean (or depend) on my own understanding. In all my ways, I will acknowledge You, because Your Word assures me that You will direct my paths (see Proverbs 3:5-6, NKJV).

My heart longs to trust You completely with everything in my life, not just my First Place plans and goals. Help me to learn how to do this more. I need You, Lord, to give me wisdom and to guide me in Your path for my life.

Notes

1. Neva Coyle, *Free to Dream* (Minneapolis, MN: Bethany House Publishers, 1990), p. 23. Used by permission.
2. Beth Moore, *Praying God's Word* (Nashville, TN: Broadman and Holman, 2000), p. 155.
3. Ibid., p. 156.
4. Ibid., p. 95.
5. Ibid., p. 133.
6. Ibid., p. 130.
7. Ibid., p. 93.

GROUP PRAYER REQUESTS   TODAY'S DATE:_____

NAME	REQUEST	RESULTS

SURRENDER FOR SUCCESS

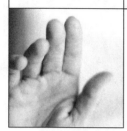

MEMORY VERSE

Love the LORD your God with all your heart and
with all your soul and with all your strength.
Deuteronomy 6:5

As we pursue our dreams, wholehearted surrender to God is essential to our success. In this week's study we will discover seven areas that greatly influence our success in life. As you read, ask God to reveal to you anyone or anything that holds more value to you than Him. Seek ways you can demonstrate your commitment to Him as your Lord, who alone is worthy of your worship and service.

DAY 1: *Our Affections and Appetites*

➤ According to Colossians 3:1-10, where are we "to set," or focus, our hearts and minds?

When Christ is our life, earthly habits and attitudes displeasing to Him must be put to death. These must be replaced with the new self.

➤ Do you have something in your life that needs to be put to death? If so, explain.

We cannot conquer the old nature in our own power. God provides a way for us to be obedient. Read again the first verse of Colossians 3. Paul stated that we "have been raised with Christ." The power of the resurrected Christ transforms us!

⟫ Consider verses 9-10 again—what is the process through which Christ helps us take off the old self?

Through the indwelling Holy Spirit, Christ renews us daily, conforming us to His image.

⟫ According to Deuteronomy 6:5 and Mark 12:30, how are we to love God?

Setting our affections on God is another way of saying we love God. Loving God enables us to overcome the temptations that have ruled us.

Where are your affections directed? Consider people, places, material possessions, even food. If your affections keep you from wholehearted surrender to God, ask Him to put to death all that comes before Him in your heart. In your prayer journal today, ask God to give you a heart that is filled with His love. Begin to memorize this week's memory verse. Use it in your prayer today.

Few things in life drive us more than our appetites. God wants us to desire something more valuable than physical food or pleasure. Jesus said, "Blessed are those who hunger and thirst for righteousness, for they will be filled" (Matthew 5:6). Surrendering both our affections and our appetites to God will help us along the road to success.

Genesis 25:29-34 tells the story of one person who let his hunger for food alter his entire future. We do not know if craving food was a habit or just an event in Esau's life. He let his desire for food control him. He took the gift of his birthright lightly. Esau's desire for food was stronger than his desire to keep his rightful inheritance.

➤ Read the following Scriptures and match each with its summary statement on the right:

_____ Psalm 63:5   a. My soul will be satisfied by You as with the richest of foods.

_____ Psalm 107:8-9   b. Jesus' food was to do His Father's will and to finish His work.

_____ Psalm 119:103   c. Jesus is the Bread of Life. Anyone who comes to Him will never hunger. Anyone who believes in Him will never thirst.

_____ Matthew 4:4   d. The words of the Lord are sweeter than honey to us.

_____ John 4:34   e. Man does not live on bread alone but on the Word of God.

_____ John 6:35   f. Crave spiritual milk so that you can grow in your salvation.

_____ 1 Peter 2:2-3   g. God satisfies our thirst and hunger with the good things of Him.

Cindy simply enjoyed good food and loved to eat! Throughout the day she found herself thinking of her next meal or snack. She enjoyed grocery shopping and planning meals. She watched gourmet food-preparation shows on television and subscribed to several food-oriented magazines. One day during worship her pastor asked, "Who or what controls you?" Cindy immediately thought of food. In fact, during the service she had been daydreaming about baking a cake after church. That day Cindy decided to give God control of her life.

Do any of the appetites of your flesh control you? It may be a lust—a hunger and thirst—for food, sex, alcohol, material possessions, power, wealth, acceptance, recognition, career or social status. Surrender it to God.

As you eat your bread exchanges today, remember that Jesus is the Bread of Life. He will nourish and satisfy your every hunger and thirst!

Father God, it is my heart's desire to love You above all else. Help me to give You control over all of my life.

Lord, put a righteous appetite for You and for Your Word in its proper place—first place—in my life! Please satisfy the longings of my soul.

DAY 2: *Our Allegiance*

Americans repeat the Pledge of Allegiance to the American flag and all it represents. However, as Christians we know we also have a higher allegiance. Today, we will be challenged to pledge allegiance to God.

Joshua followed the example of Moses in giving God priority in his life. In Joshua 24:14-15, he urged the Israelites to renew their covenant with God.

≫ What did Joshua tell the people to throw away? What choice did they need to make?

≫ If we don't choose to serve God, what is our only other choice?

≫ What do you need to throw away that is keeping you from putting God first in your life?

In Matthew 6:24, Jesus cautioned us against trying to serve two masters. By definition, a master is whatever or whoever is in control. If we call Jesus "Lord," He must be our only master. Paul often called himself the servant of Christ (see Romans 1:1). We, too, are called to serve Christ.

➤ According to Ephesians 6:7, what attitude should a Christian servant have?

When we serve with our whole heart, holding nothing back from God, He rewards us for every good action (see Ephesians 6:8). If you have never made the choice to serve God, prayerfully make that choice today.

 Holy God, help me to put my trust in You and to be completely loyal to You. I choose to serve You alone and to surrender my will to Yours, because this is essential to become all You desire for me.

DAY 3: *Our Attitudes and Actions*

Our attitudes influence and determine our actions. Both attitudes and actions determine our success. God calls us to surrender our attitudes and actions to Him.

Consider your attitudes as you read Romans 8:5-9.

➤ What is the result of the mind controlled by the sinful nature?

➤ What is the result of the mind controlled by the Spirit?

➤ If the Spirit of God lives in you, who controls you?

Consider your actions as you read Psalm 1:1-3.

➤ Draw a line to connect the actions avoided by the person who is surrendered to God.

Does not walk	in the way of sinners.
Does not stand	in the counsel of the wicked.
Does not sit	in the seat of mockers.

➤ Draw a line to connect the actions of the person surrendered to God.

Meditates	in whatever he does.
Yields	in the law of the Lord.
Prospers	on God's law day and night.
Delights	fruit and does not wither in whatever he does.

➤ How do your attitudes and actions contribute to your success or lack of success in following the First Place program?

	HELPFUL	NOT HELPFUL
Attitudes		
Actions		

Cooperate with God as He brings your attitudes and actions in line with His will. Take time to review your memory verses and ask the Lord to speak to you through the verses you are learning.

Dear God, I choose to surrender my attitudes and actions to You. "Create in me a pure heart, O God, and renew a steadfast spirit within me. Restore to me the joy of your salvation and grant me a willing spirit, to sustain me" (Psalm 51:10,12).

DAY 4: *Our Anxieties and Answers*

Often Cindy found herself paralyzed by fear. What if something happened to her? Who would take care of her children? What if a major medical expense wiped out her meager savings? In times of fear, she brought her concerns to God. Like Cindy, we need to wholeheartedly surrender our fears to the Lord. He invites us to trust Him.

➤ According to Philippians 4:6-7, what are we to do with our anxieties? Check one of the following:

☐ Fret ☐ Solve the problem ourselves

☐ Despair ☐ Pray

➤ After reading 1 Peter 5:7, fill in the blanks:

Cast _____ your _____ on Him because He _____ for you.

➤ In Mark 4:35-41, what was Jesus able to do (v. 39)?

➤ What did Jesus ask the disciples in verse 40?

Jesus called on the disciples to exercise faith. Faith requires us to trust God during the storms of life. We develop faith through Bible study, prayer and obedience.

Do you have fears or anxieties? Are you afraid of failing in First Place?

Do other worries cause fear to haunt you? If so, cast each one on your Savior and surrender them to His care. He will replace your fears with His peace. He has the answer to your every concern.

Human nature inclines us to trust in our own wisdom or the counsel of others. God wants us to look to Him for the answers to every situation and circumstance. When we need answers, we should rely on Him.

➤ After reading Proverbs 3:5-6, put a T (for true) or an F (for false) in each blank.

_____ God instructs me to trust Him completely for guidance.

_____ I can trust in my own wisdom and understanding.

_____ God will direct my paths when I acknowledge Him in all I do.

➤ In your own words, summarize the teachings found in 2 Corinthians 9:8; Ephesians 3:20-21 and Philippians 4:19.

➤ In the past, when trying to lose weight or solve other health concerns, where have you looked for answers?

God's answer to your weight-health problem may be the First Place program. He can use your First Place group leaders and members to provide guidance as you seek His will together. Trust God to provide the right answers for your life regarding your need to lose or manage your weight and improve your fitness level.

Father, I trust that You have the perfect answer for every aspect of my life. When You give me Your answers, help me to follow Your instructions.

DAY 5: *Our Adoration*

Wholehearted surrender manifests itself most clearly and sweetly in adoration. Nothing deserves our adoration more than our Savior, who loved us so much that He willingly died on the cross in our place. A life completely surrendered to Him will know the highest of joys and contentment.

⟫ According to Mark 14:3-9, why did the woman anoint Jesus with perfume?

⟫ Describe the perfume's value.

⟫ What was the reaction of the people?

⟫ What was Jesus' response?

⟫ How will the woman be remembered?

When you present a gift to someone you love, you want it to be the very best you can give, in top-notch condition and packaged attractively. You may have sacrificed to present a pleasing gift. In Romans 12:1, Paul urges us "in view of God's mercy, to offer [our] bodies as living sacrifices, holy and pleasing to God—this is [our] spiritual act of worship." Sacrifices to God are to be pure, unblemished. Do you desire to present your body in the best possible condition, whatever the cost? What are you doing to make your body the best it can be? Presenting our bodies as an acceptable sacrifice is an act of worship.

Is there anyone you adore more than Jesus? Anything you cherish or hold on to more than your salvation? You need to surrender yourself completely, putting Him in first place.

 Father God, help me surrender whatever keeps me from adoring You above all else. I offer You a life wholeheartedly surrendered.

DAY 6: *Reflections*

Surrender is often a very hard thing to do. For those who are strong willed, fiercely independent or too proud, it can be an enormous challenge to surrender at all—let alone wholeheartedly! Without question, this week's study most likely challenges all of us in one area of our lives or another.

Surrender is usually perceived as giving up, giving in, of doing what we don't want to do. However, when we follow the example of Christ, who surrendered completely to the Father, surrender means giving over and beginning anew. As we begin to turn over everything in our lives to the Father in Christlike surrender, He opens new avenues and paths that we have never seen before. The Lord can then replace our old habits and desires with new Christlike conduct, desires, direction and goals.

➣ Of the following, check those areas in your life that still need to be surrendered:

☐	My affections	☐	My actions
☐	My appetites	☐	My anxieties
☐	My allegiance	☐	My answers
☐	My attitudes	☐	My adoration

➤ What impact would surrender in any of these areas have on your ability to be successful in following the First Place commitments?

➤ How would it change your behavior each day?

➤ What impact would wholehearted surrender have on your relationship with God?

➤ How would it change your behavior each day?

Father God, I acknowledge that I have struggles and difficulties in giving these areas over to You. Please help me with this. I praise You for the grace You've given me in those areas that are not difficult to surrender.

Jesus, according to Your Word, if I truly desire to come after You, I must deny myself and take up my cross and follow You (see Luke 9:23).[1] Help me, Lord, to let go of my right to have things my own way. Help me choose to surrender to Your ways—to Your will for my life. Teach me to follow You more each day.

Father, Your Word assures me that it is You who works in me to will and to act according to Your good purpose (see Philippians 2:13).[2] It is my heart's desire, Lord, to be led by Your Spirit and to live according to Your will, even though at times my old sin nature fights against me. Help me to surrender fully to You. Help me to follow Jesus' example and give everything over to You.

My Father, You are the Lord my God. I desire to love You, listen to Your voice and hold fast to You, for You, Lord, are my life (see Deuteronomy 30:20).[3]

Awesome God, Your Word says that knowing Christ Jesus as my Lord is so wonderful that I can consider everything a loss in comparison to the surpassing greatness of that relationship. Help me to consider as rubbish anything that I have to lay down in order to gain more knowledge and a more abiding presence of Christ (see Philippians 3:8).[4]

DAY 7: *Reflections*

The title of this week's lesson is "Surrender for Success." In order to know true success, the kind of success God wants us to experience, we need to surrender in each of the different areas discussed this week, as well as any others that God chooses to reveal to us.

Perhaps God wants us to realize that anything we hold on to, anything that we are unable or unwilling to give over to Him, is likely holding on to us. In other words, the very thing we hold with a tight grip and do not surrender to God actually holds a tight grip on us. This grip prevents us from experiencing all that God wants to give us. If we would just let go and free our hearts and lives, we could then receive what the Lord has planned for us. Being willing to let go, surrendering every aspect of our lives to the Lord, enables us to receive God's plan for success in our lives. Are there things you are still holding on to that are causing you to be a captive? Letting go will mean your freedom through Christ.

You may be thinking: *Okay, I realize I need to surrender wholeheartedly—to give over every aspect of my life to God, but how do I do that? It is so hard!* Yes, surrender may be difficult. To a great extent it requires us to deny our own will, our personal wishes, and sometimes our feelings (for example: bitterness, anger, envy, jealousy). We struggle against our old nature, the old self discussed in Days 1 and 6. Surrender involves humility and submission to God; we need to humbly submit and relinquish our will in order to surrender to God. We can learn a great deal about how to surrender our will from the example of our Lord and Savior, Jesus Christ.

Recall the words of Jesus as He prayed in the garden shortly before

His crucifixion. Jesus prayed and honestly poured out His heart, but He ultimately said, "not my will, but yours be done" (Luke 22:42). In humble submission, Jesus not only surrendered His will, but He also surrendered *every* aspect of His life to the Father.

Surrendering our lives to God is vital to our dreams and goals becoming reality. As we give God control of every aspect of our lives and humbly submit to Him, we will discover that the glorious pathway to success is now open to us.

➤ Review this list of the First Place commitments and check any that are difficult for you—especially any that involve a need for you to surrender your will.

☐ Attendance   ☐ Encouragement

☐ Bible study   ☐ Live-It plan

☐ Prayer   ☐ Commitment Record

☐ Scripture reading   ☐ Exercise

☐ Memory verse

When we pray as Jesus did, God will give us the strength we need to surrender every aspect of our lives to Him. He will also provide the strength we need to accomplish His will.

Lord, according to Your Word, the key to not gratifying the desires of the sinful nature is to live by the Spirit (see Galatians 5:16). Teach me to live by Your Spirit, Lord.[5] Help me to surrender my will to Yours—in every area of my life.

Glorious Lord, "I have been crucified with Christ and I no longer live, but Christ lives in me. The life I live in the body, I live by faith in the Son of God, who loved me and gave himself for me" (Galatians 2:20).[6] Help me not to forget this great truth!

I praise You, Lord, that because Christ lives in me, I have the power to surrender to You daily. With Your power in me, I can learn to follow and live by Your Word. I can also carry out the First Place commitments—not in a legalistic way as if to gain favor with You or others, but from a heart that desires to please You. I want to live as best I can according to the spirit and intent of the First Place program and Your Word.

I know I can't be perfect in this—Jesus is the only perfect one—but I can live for You with Your power in me.

Lord, "you are my God, earnestly I seek you; my soul thirsts for you . . . in a dry and weary land where there is no water. I have seen you in the sanctuary and beheld your power and your glory. Because your love is better than life, my lips will glorify you. I will praise you as long as I live, and in your name I will lift up my hands. My soul will be satisfied as with the richest of foods; with singing lips my mouth will praise you" (Psalm 63:1-5). Father, making a decision to seek Your will, above all else, helps me to begin to surrender my life to You. O Lord, please walk with me on this journey because I need You.

Notes
1. Beth Moore, *Praying God's Word* (Nashville, TN: Broadman and Holman, 2000), p. 165.
2. Ibid., p. 144.
3. Ibid., p. 22.
4. Ibid., p. 144.
5. Ibid., p. 162.
6. Ibid., p. 49.

GROUP PRAYER REQUESTS   TODAY'S DATE:_____

NAME	REQUEST	RESULTS

DRESS FOR SUCCESS

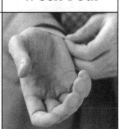

MEMORY VERSE

*Put on the full armor of God so that you can take
your stand against the devil's schemes.*

Ephesians 6:11

In the business world, Cindy found that dress plays a major role in deter-
mining success. Projecting the right image can make a great difference
when applying for a position, conducting business meetings or working in
sales. Did you know that Christians have a dress code for success? In this
week's study we will discover seven wardrobe essentials for Christians
seeking to accomplish their goals.

DAY 1: *The Belt of Truth*

Truthfulness is an essential part of the Christian's wardrobe. Unfortunately,
many in our society have developed their own standards of right and wrong.
Their standards are not founded on God's truth. In Ephesians 6:10-18, the
belt of truth in the full armor of God is described as our first defense against
Satan. A soldier's belt held all the other garments in place. God's truth will
hold all the rest of our armor in place as we face our enemy, Satan.

➤ According to Ephesians 6:10-18, against whom do we wrestle?

➤ Why should we put on God's armor?

⫸ In the following lists, cross out the words that are the opposite of truth:

Sincerity	Dishonesty
Lies	Trustworthiness
Evil	Integrity
Falsehood	Faithfulness
Dependability	Honesty
Virtue	Justice
Scheming	Purity

⫸ According to Titus 1:1-12, can God be trusted?

⫸ Is God faithful and true?

⫸ According to John 14:1, can Jesus be trusted?

God's very nature is truthfulness.

⫸ In John 8:42-45, how does Jesus describe Satan?

⫸ What is Satan's native language?

⫸ Can Satan be trusted?

What lies does Satan tell you? Does he try to tell you that you are a failure, that you will never lose weight or that you will never reach your goals? Does Satan try to deceive you and make you doubt God's Word? Take time to begin learning the memory verse for this week.

 Father God, I ask You to deafen my ears to Satan's lies and help me to hear Your voice.

Lord God, help me to refute Satan's lies with Your belt of truth. Thank You, mighty God, that I am a child of Yours, my King!

DAY 2: *The Breastplate of Righteousness; the Gospel of Peace*

In addition to the belt of truth, the Christian wardrobe includes the breast-plate of righteousness. Much like a modern-day bulletproof vest worn by a law enforcement officer, a breastplate was worn by a soldier to guard the vital organs, especially the heart. As soldiers of the King, we must wear the breastplate of righteousness to protect our hearts from Satan. An unguard-ed heart gets us into trouble.

Righteousness is a gift of God's grace to those who receive salvation through Jesus Christ. Jesus' sinless life covers our sin so that God sees only the righteousness of Christ when He looks at you and me (see Romans 3:20-24). When we are right with God, we do what is right, but those who live a lifestyle of sin are of the devil (see 1 John 3:7-8).

➤ Proverbs 4:23 warns us to_____because it

   is the_____of life.

➤ After reading Luke 6:45, in your own words explain the contrast between the two hearts described by Jesus.

As you get dressed today, figuratively dress yourself in your bulletproof vest, your breastplate of righteousness. In your prayer journal, thank God for the crimson blood that was shed by Jesus to give you a gloriously radi-ant, spotless, white robe of righteousness to guard your heart. Only His righteousness can defeat the enemy.

After urging us to put on the belt of truth and the breastplate of right-eousness, Paul also emphasized the need for the soldier's feet to be prepared. What did he mean when he instructed us to have our "feet fitted with the readiness that comes from the gospel of peace" (Ephesians 6:15)? One busy evening, God used the simple, everyday events of Cindy's life to help her understand.

Following a busy day at work, Cindy was making a new recipe for dinner. She reached into the cupboard only to discover she was out of a key ingredient. Later, she searched for a shirt in her closet, only to find it in the laundry pile she had failed to wash the night before. And shortly before bedtime, Cindy's daughter needed her to rush out to get supplies to complete a project due the next morning at school. As we study this piece of the armor, we discover God's challenge is to be prepared.

In Paul's day, wearing sandals was a sign of a person's being equipped and ready to move. Christians who are fitted with the footwear of the gospel of peace are ready to share the good news of Jesus with others.

➽ How are Isaiah 52:7 and Romans 10:15 related to Ephesians 6:15?

➽ According to 2 Timothy 4:1-2, when are we to be prepared?

➽ What are we to be prepared to do?

➽ What should be our approach?

➽ Why are we to be prepared?

Jesus has provided peace with God for us. We have been forgiven our past sin and restored to new life in Christ. The gospel of peace is our firm footing and gives us balance. Is there anything more wonderful than the serenity of soul and the calmness of spirit that the gospel of peace gives?

Psalm 119:165 says, "Great peace have they who love your law, and nothing can make them stumble." As you grow spiritually and God manifests Himself to you more each day through Bible study, Scripture memorization and prayer, the peace of God will grow in your heart. As it does, observe the impact on your eating and the other commitments. The peace of God satisfies the soul like no food can. As you experience His peace in your life, be prepared to share the source of that peace with others.

 Lord, as I prepare for today, I'm grateful for the armor You've supplied for me. I put on the breastplate of righteousness to protect my heart. I strap on my combat boots—the gospel of peace. By Your grace I will be ready to stand firm and take action in the daily struggle to say yes to You and no to Satan.

Father God, please bring to my mind someone who needs to hear the good news of Jesus Christ from me!

DAY 3: *The Shield of Faith; the Helmet of Salvation*

Consider Ephesians 6:16 again. The shield of faith is our belief and trust in God. Satan cannot get past this shield, but he can throw fiery darts all around it and try to create havoc in our lives. A soldier holds his shield on his arm, so he can readily move it to deflect arrows that can come from every direction. Hold up your shield of faith at all times.

➤ Hebrews 11:1 describes faith as _____ of what

we hope for and_____of what we cannot see.

Faith requires us to believe in God, even when we cannot see how the situation will turn out. The heroes of the faith listed in Hebrews 11 were commended because they obeyed God, often without living to see the fulfillment of God's promises (see Hebrews 11:39).

➤ Hebrews 11:6 says without faith it is_____

to please God.

➤ In Daniel 3:15-18, was the faith of Shadrach, Meshach and Abednego dependent on whether or not God rescued them?

    ☐ Yes   ☐ No

➤ What impact did holding up their shield of faith have on the king (see Daniel 3:28-30)?

The account of Shadrach, Meshach and Abednego reminds us not to place our faith in anyone or anything but God. Ask God to help you recognize any areas of your life where you worship other gods and put your faith in something or someone other than God Almighty.

Do you have the shield of faith? If so, boldly hold it up and let God be your shield against Satan's attacks. If not, choose to place your faith and hope in Jesus now and receive the only shield of protection you will ever need. As you pray, tell Him you accept His invitation today.

With shield in hand to protect his upper body, a soldier going into battle would also need to protect his head with a strong, dependable helmet. As you face life's battles, be sure to wear your helmet of salvation to protect your mind from Satan's control.

The helmet of salvation protects the sound mind that God gives us. In 1 Thessalonians 5:5-8, Paul encouraged us to be self-controlled and to put on the helmet of salvation. Before we can share the message of salvation with others, we must experience it for ourselves. Salvation comes as a free gift to those who trust Jesus as Savior and Lord.

➤ Read the following Scriptures and match them with the correct summary statements:

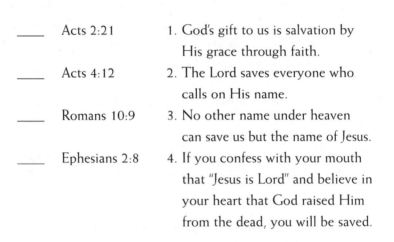

_____	Acts 2:21	1. God's gift to us is salvation by His grace through faith.
_____	Acts 4:12	2. The Lord saves everyone who calls on His name.
_____	Romans 10:9	3. No other name under heaven can save us but the name of Jesus.
_____	Ephesians 2:8	4. If you confess with your mouth that "Jesus is Lord" and believe in your heart that God raised Him from the dead, you will be saved.

➤ Write a summary statement about how we receive the helmet of salvation.

Salvation puts us on the path to true success. If you have surrendered your life to Jesus Christ, take time to thank Him for His salvation. If you have not received Him as Lord and Savior, pray right now. Confess to Him that you are a sinner. Tell Him you are sorry for your sins and choose to follow His ways. Call upon Him to come into your life as Savior and Lord. Commit your life to Him in gratitude. Pray for Christ's light to shine through you as you put on your helmet of salvation. Thank Him for His

gift of salvation. If you have prayed this prayer, share your decision with
your group leader, a pastor or a Christian friend.

 Lord, help me to make good decisions each day as I continue
to pursue the plans and goals You have given me. Please protect my mind from Satan's attacks and guard the decision I
made last week to surrender to You.

DAY 4: *The Sword of the Spirit*

The sword of the Spirit is the only offensive weapon in our wardrobe.
Our sword is the Word of God. We penetrate the devil's strongholds
when we effectively use God's Word to defeat him.

Consider Matthew 4:1-11; Jesus is our example in winning the battle
against Satan.

>> In his attack on Jesus, what were the three temptations Satan used?

>> How did Jesus respond in each case? What was His weapon?

>> How did Satan ultimately respond to the weapon Jesus used?

Jesus had memorized each of the Scriptures. Psalm 119:11 reminds
us to hide God's Word in our hearts that we might not sin against Him.
Have you memorized this week's Scripture verse? If not, do so now.

>> Try to write this week's memory verse without looking it up or refer-
ring to the first page of this lesson.

Read the following Scriptures and select one or more to record in your prayer journal. These verses will be a source of help and strength when you face the enemy: Psalm 119:105; Colossians 3:16; 2 Timothy 3:16; Hebrews 4:12.

 Lord God, I know the Holy Bible is my sword. Help me to actively fight the devil's schemes with my offensive weapon, rather than merely dodging his arrows with my shield held high in defense.

God, help me win victories by meditating on Your Word.

DAY 5: *Staying Alert*

Cindy took a defensive-driving course. The instructor stressed the importance of staying alert to what other drivers were doing. "Never let down your guard," he said. "Anticipating what may happen may in fact keep it from happening." God's Word instructs us to watch carefully and be alert. The key to staying alert, according to Ephesians 6:18, is prayer. This verse also tells us to pray in the Spirit.

➤ After reading Romans 8:26, describe the role of the Spirit in our prayers.

➤ According to 1 Peter 5:8, we are to be alert to what danger?

Staying alert involves being aware of the devil's schemes and being determined to keep from falling victim to him. Even Paul recognized his need for prayer and coveted the prayers of his fellow believers. "Pray also for me," said Paul, "that whenever I open my mouth, words may be given me so that I will fearlessly make known the mystery of the gospel" (Ephesians 6:19). Ask God to bring someone to mind who needs your prayers today.

Your First Place group meetings are a great place to learn to pray for others.

➤ How have the prayers of others in the group been an encouragement to you?

➤ Whom will you encourage through prayer today?

➤ Do you have a specific quiet time each day? If so, when is it and where?

➤ What is the instruction found in 1 Thessalonians 5:17?

➤ How can you maintain communication with God during your day?

➤ Consider Ephesians 6:18 again; do you pray about everything or only the big things in life?

Staying alert through prayer can help you with your First Place commitments.

➤ Indicate one or more of your commitments whose fulfillment requires God's help.

Learning to stay alert and on guard to defend against an enemy's attack is essential for any well-trained soldier. Learning to pray and rely on God's power to help us stand against the devil requires a continued attitude of prayer, compelling us to stay in close communication with God throughout each day.

The familiar hymn "In the Garden" reminds us how very much our Savior desires to spend time with us. He wants to walk with us and talk with us. Tarry in the garden today as long as you can.

Mighty God, I ask that You give me the strength and power I need to stand firm and resist the attacks of Satan. Thank You that for those of us who wear the armor of God, nothing can defeat us or separate us from the victory we have in You, our resurrected Savior, Jesus Christ.

DAY 6: *Reflections*

In this week's study, we learned about the armor of God, the wardrobe of a soldier of Christ. Success in the battle against the enemy demands that we be equipped and properly dressed for battle. Life on this earth presents many challenges, trials and tribulations for every human being. For the Christian, these can easily become the battleground the devil chooses for his attacks. The devil's ultimate goal is to defeat God's children—he will use anything he can to do so.

The following list presents examples of battles, strongholds, challenges or difficulties people sometimes experience:

Abuse	Alcohol	Anger or hatred	Bitterness
Critical, or judgmental, attitude	Death of loved one	Depression	Disappointment
Divorce	Drug addiction	Eating disorders	Envy or jealousy
Family quarrels	Fear or anxiety	Gambling	Greed
Hunger	Illness or disease	Lack of education	Lonelinesss
Loss of job	Lust	Natural disasters	Physical handicaps
Political oppression	Pornography	Poverty	Prejudice
Pride	Religious persecution	Unforgiveness	Weight management

Contemplate the kinds of weapons people sometimes rely on when faced with strongholds or battles—weapons such as counselors, willpower and so on. The world's weapons may at times offer help, but deep strongholds and battles require more. Victory is assured for those who depend on God's weaponry. Second Corinthians 10:4 says, "The weapons we fight with are not the weapons of the world. On the contrary, they have divine power to demolish strongholds."

Continue to study and memorize Scripture. Review the previous week's memory verses. As you do this, you will build a great arsenal of God's Word in heart and mind and you will be ready in the day of battle. Practice drawing your sword of the Spirit by using the Scripture prayers, or select a Scripture on your own and use personal pronouns wherever appropriate.

Lord God, You are my stronghold in time of trouble. Help me and deliver me; deliver me from the wicked and save me because I take refuge in You (see Psalm 37:39-40).[1]

Father, Your Word instructs me to put on the full armor of God so that I can take my stand against the devil's schemes. For my struggle is not against flesh and blood, but against the rulers, against the authorities, against the powers of this dark world and against the spiritual forces of evil in the heavenly realms. Therefore, help me to put on the full armor of God so that when the day of evil comes I will be able to stand my ground (see Ephesians 6:10-13). Don't ever let me forget that I have a very real enemy who wants me in bondage. Help me to discern his schemes and take my stand against him in the power of Your Spirit.[2]

Father, according to Your Word, in this world I will have trouble, but I am to take heart! You have overcome the world (see John 16:33).[3] Therefore, I will trust in You to help me overcome my struggles. Empower me to overcome temptations by learning to quote Your Word, just as Jesus did when Satan tempted Him in the wilderness. Help me to memorize the weekly Scripture verses, Lord. It isn't always easy for me, but when I encounter trouble, I want to draw on the power of Your Word to defeat the enemy.

DAY 7: *Reflections*

Now that you have learned about the essential wardrobe every Christian needs, reflect again on two points covered in this week's study: self-control and staying alert. In 1 Thessalonians 5:5-8, we were urged to stay alert and pray. It seems that a connection exists between self-control and staying alert. Perhaps a self-controlled life tends to be more on guard and therefore less vulnerable to Satan's attacks.

Take a few moments to consider times when self-control may have had a *positive* impact on your life and other times when a *lack* of self-control may have had a *negative* impact on your life. You may want to record your thoughts in your prayer journal. Think about your answer to this question: *Am I currently out of control, or am I self-controlled?* Being self-controlled is not something we do out of our own strength or willpower. Recall Galatians 5:22-23; along with several other qualities, self-control is listed as a fruit of the Spirit. It develops in us as we nurture the presence of the Holy Spirit in our hearts, as we allow Him to control our lives more each day.

Living a self-controlled, prayer-filled life and dressing in the armor of God can impact all we do and make it possible for us to live in triumph and victory by the power of Christ. Faithfully living the life God has called us to live can affect our degree of success in our work, in First Place, in relationships with others, in our Christian growth, in defeating anything that binds us.

As you move on to a new week, remember to be alert to the devil's schemes, faithfully wear your armor and firmly hold your sword—the Word of God.

 Father God, You have said we are to be sober and vigilant because our adversary the devil, like a roaring lion, walks around seeking whom he may devour (see 1 Peter 5:8). Thank You for teaching me through this lesson how to prepare for encounters with the enemy and how to be alert and vigilant.

Thank You as well, Lord, for Your promise which says that Your eyes range throughout the earth to strengthen those whose hearts are fully committed to You (see 2 Chronicles 16:9). Keep Your eyes on me, Lord, and help me to have a heart that is fully committed to You.

Father God, deliver me from the lion's mouth just as You did the apostle Paul. Rescue me from every evil attack and bring me safely to Your heavenly kingdom. To You be glory for ever and ever. Amen (see 2 Timothy 4:17-18).[4]

Lord God, You are the great I AM. This is Your name *forever* (see Exodus 3:14-15)! My enemy cannot begin to stand against You.[5] You are my hope, Lord; I am depending on You.

I will sing to You, Lord, for You are highly exalted. The horse and its rider You have hurled into the sea! You, Lord, are my strength and my song; You have become my salvation. You are my God and I will praise You. You, Lord, are a warrior! The Lord is Your name (see Exodus 15:1-3).[6]

Notes

1. Beth Moore, *Praying God's Word* (Nashville, TN: Broadman and Holman, 2000), p. 320.
2. Ibid., p. 144.
3. Ibid., p. 326.
4. Ibid., p. 330.
5 Ibid., p. 312.
6. Ibid.

GROUP PRAYER REQUESTS   TODAY'S DATE:_____

NAME	REQUEST	RESULTS

KEYS TO SUCCESS

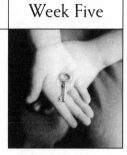

MEMORY VERSE

His divine power has given us everything we need for life and godliness through our knowledge of him who called us by his own glory and goodness.

2 Peter 1:3

Have you ever lost your keys and frantically searched for them? When you lose the keys to your home or car, you might experience feelings of fear and frustration. Why? Because keys give you access to important places, and when you lose that access, you can feel helpless. In your search for the keys to success, God has provided several that can one by one open the locked doors in your life. In this week's study, God's Word will help you locate the keys that unlock the doorways to success.

DAY 1: *Commitment and Effort; Obedience and Blessings*

The first keys to success are commitment and effort. When you make a sincere commitment to something, you must then put every effort into accomplishing your commitment.

➤ According to Proverbs 16:3, what must we do first when making plans?

➤ According to 1 Kings 8:61, what must be fully committed to God?

Have you made a sincere commitment to the Lord regarding the First Place program and the plans and goals the Lord has led you to make? If not, perhaps you would consider telling God you have a heart that is willing to be made fully committed.

Make a note of today's date in the margin and ask God to keep your heart open to Him and to empower you to honor your commitment to Him.

➤ According to 2 Peter 1:3, what has God given us?

➤ Place a check beside each of the following qualities you have committed to adding to your faith:

☐ Knowledge	☐ Goodness
☐ Self-control	☐ Love
☐ Godliness	☐ Brotherly kindness
☐ Perseverance	

In your prayer journal today, ask God to help you make every effort to add to your faith the seven qualities listed in 2 Peter 1:5-7. Review the nine First Place commitments in the following chart. Check any commitments that need more effort on your part. Make a note on the chart regarding what action (effort) you will take this week to keep each commitment you checked. As you pray today, ask God to help you follow through.

Commitments	Actions/Efforts
☐ Attendance	
☐ Prayer	
☐ Scripture reading	

Commitments	Actions/Efforts
☐ Memory verse	
☐ Bible study	
☐ Live-It plan	
☐ Commitment Record	
☐ Encouragement	
☐ Exercise	

Keeping commitments requires obedience. Does the word "obedience" sting your ears? Our culture glorifies independence and instant gratification. We do not want anyone telling us what to do or what not to do, what to eat or what not to eat! Obedience, however, is the key that opens the door to God's blessings. If we want to receive all the blessings He has in store for us, we must learn to obey God. The keys of obedience and blessings work in partnership with the keys of commitment and effort.

Write Deuteronomy 7:9 in your prayer journal. Circle God's promise and underline His conditions.

➤ After reading Deuteronomy 28:1-14, list at least three of the blessings of obedience that God promises.

➤ Are there still blessings for obedience today?

    ☐ Yes   ☐ No

➤ What are some of the blessings of obedience in the First Place program?

➤ In which areas of First Place are you currently obedient to God's direction and instruction?

➤ Are there consequences for disobedience?

    ☐ Yes   ☐ No

➤ What blessings of obedience have you experienced as a result of First Place?

When we know what we need to do for healthy bodies and don't do it, we hurt ourselves. Disobedience robs us of blessings. Every day wear the armor of God you studied last week to help you in the daily battles you face. Review your memory verse and ask God to help you develop an obedient heart. You can anticipate showers of heavenly blessings.

Father, I've recorded the actions that I will take this week to keep each commitment I've checked. Please help me follow through.

DAY 2: *Honesty and Integrity*

Cindy struggled to be totally honest when completing a First Place Commitment Record. She wanted to turn in a perfect record. Often she was tempted to give up keeping her Commitment Record because she had missing exchanges—or worse, went over on exchanges or failed to measure exchanges at all! She didn't want anyone to know that she did not follow the Live-It plan perfectly, nor did she want anyone to know when she had other imperfect commitments!

However difficult, personal honesty and integrity are critical keys to success in all areas of First Place and in everyday life.

➣ According to Proverbs 11:1-6, what does the Lord abhor?

➣ What does the Lord delight in?

➣ What is the benefit to those who live with integrity?

➣ What is the way of those who are righteous and blameless, and what becomes of the wicked?

Evaluate your honesty by answering each of the following questions:

➤ Do you weigh and measure your foods whenever possible?

☐ Yes   ☐ No

➤ Do you level that tablespoon of margarine or peanut butter?

☐ Yes   ☐ No

➤ Do you record everything you eat?

☐ Yes   ☐ No

➤ Do you accurately record your exercise time, distance and/or number of repetitions?

☐ Yes   ☐ No

➤ Do you pray daily?

☐ Yes   ☐ No

➤ Do you complete your Bible study daily?

☐ Yes   ☐ No

As you read James 1:21-25, look into your heart's mirror.

➤ What would need to change in your life right now in order to demonstrate honesty and integrity?

Cindy needed to look deep inside; she needed to understand that honesty and integrity begin with being honest with herself and with God, the One who already knows the facts anyway. Cindy needed to change her focus from being concerned about disappointing her leader or her classmates and to change her heart attitude by not lying to herself about what she was eating or about how well she was keeping her commitments. She needed to accept that she could not be perfect and remember that Jesus is the only perfect One. She needed to realize the great value, divine blessing and personal integrity that are found in striving for excellence, not perfection. Cindy decided to enlist the help of the keys of commitment and effort by sincerely doing the best she could and then honestly recording her eating and commitments for the week. The words of the psalmist provided Cindy with a great promise from God and encouraged her to change. Psalm 41:12 says, "In my integrity you uphold me and set me in your presence forever."

Honesty is your friend and ally. Jesus declared, "I am the truth" (see John 14:6). He will guide you, uphold you and allow you the privilege of dwelling in the sanctuary of our God.

Lord Jesus, I can wear the breastplate of righteousness today with gratitude to You, the One who paid the price for it.

Holy God, help me to be a person of integrity and thereby honor You.

DAY 3: *Wisdom and Understanding*

God's Word declares that wisdom will be granted to all who seek it (see James 1:5). As you study today, consider how wisdom and understanding can help you obtain success.

➤ Write the verse from James 1:5 in your prayer journal. Underline God's instructions on how to attain wisdom and circle the word that describes how God gives wisdom to those who ask.

➤ Contrast the two different kinds of people described in Proverbs 17:24.

≫ Contrast the two different kinds of people described in Proverbs 23:19-21.

≫ After reading Proverbs 3:13-18, list the benefits of wisdom and understanding that you want to claim for your life.

In reading Proverbs 19:20, consider what help and wisdom you need in following the First Place program. For example, is the food plan or label reading confusing to you? Have you understood how to take your training heart rate or why you need to drink so much water? Do you find Scripture memory difficult? Do your emotions impact your eating or whether or not you exercise? Be willing to seek wisdom from others when God places them in your path.

≫ Write questions you might want to ask your group leader and members.

In prayer, pour out the needs of your heart and ask God for the wisdom you need.

Father God, I ask You to graciously and generously give me wisdom and understanding. I praise You for these keys as I treasure and guard them carefully.

DAY 4: *Courage and Strength; Support and Encouragement*

Taking a new path or direction in life frequently requires a great measure of courage and strength, as well as support and encouragement along the way. God told the children of Israel not to be afraid as they prepared to cross the Jordan River into the Promised Land. When we cross the rivers in our path to the promised land of success that God has for us, we do not need to be anxious or afraid.

🙡 After reading the words of Moses in Deuteronomy 31:1-8, copy verse 6 and then underline God's command and circle God's promise.

🙡 Describe both the challenge and the promise found in 2 Chronicles 32:7-8.

🙡 Identify an anxiety or fear you have that keeps you from fully experiencing the success God wants for you.

🙡 What must happen in order to alleviate that concern?

Ask God to give you the courage and strength you need to cross the Jordan Rivers in your life. Keep your eyes on the One who will go ahead of you and lead you into your promised land. He will destroy your enemies as you keep His commands. Praise Him, for He is your *Jehovah-Nissi*—your banner of victory.

Developing the keys of courage and strength without depending on God as your source could lead to a haughty, I-don't-need-anybody spirit. Regardless of how self-reliant and independent we may want to be, every human being needs support and encouragement. When Cindy went through her painful separation and divorce, the support and encouragement she felt from God were her lifelines. God also gave her a tremendous support system of family, friends in Christ and First Place group members. Their love and prayers helped her continue on the path of success.

In 2 Thessalonians 2:16-17, Paul says the love and the grace of Jesus Christ and God our Father encourage and strengthen us.

➼ Give an example of God's love in your life.

➼ Give an example of God's grace in your life.

In Philemon 7, Paul affirmed Philemon as an encourager.

➼ Give an example of how a Christian brother or sister has refreshed your heart.

➼ Write Isaiah 40:29-31 in your own words.

➼ In what areas do you need God's support and encouragement right now?

➼ Name someone to whom you feel led to offer words of encouragement and support. When and how might you do so?

Father God, I depend on You to supply the courage and strength I need each day. I ask You to empower me to succeed, thereby increasing my faith in You as I encounter each new challenge.

I praise You for Your encouragement and support. I thank You that praising You always reminds me of Your goodness all over again, and it increases my joy as I look for ways to serve You and others each day.

DAY 5: *Patience and Fortitude*

Losing weight, getting a college degree, maturing as a Christian—all take time. We must be patient with ourselves and with the process. The amount of time needed to accomplish our goals varies for each individual. The keys of patience and fortitude enable us to enjoy the process rather than allowing it to frustrate us.

Having patience does not mean sitting and passively waiting, without any questioning or intense feelings. Biblical patience has to do with trust. Do we really believe God is there, providing a way when no way seems possible? The biblical story of Job reminds us that when the world seems to fall apart, when we pray and wonder if God has really heard us, God is there. Job never received all the answers he was seeking, but he did learn a great deal about trusting God.

➤ In Job 42:1-2, what comfort do you find?

➤ According to Daniel 10:1-12, when did God hear Daniel's prayer?

➤ When did Daniel receive the answer to his prayer?

≫ What did God's messenger commend Daniel for doing?

Holy Lord, please help me in my struggle with impatience. Give me grace to wait with patience. Keep my mind open to understanding and my heart humble before You.

Father, help me to depend on You as I progress along the pathway to success.

DAY 6: *Reflections*

In this week's study we have discovered various keys that will help us on the path to success. Our key ring is full of many necessary and important keys. But does your key ring feel a bit too heavy? Are you carrying any unnecessary keys that could be weighing you down—old keys that could hinder your progress? Consider what these unnecessary keys might be: indifference and laziness, disobedience and rebellion, pride and arrogance, dishonesty and deceitfulness, foolishness and ignorance, jealousy and envy, impatience and weakness, sarcasm and negativism, or others. Allow God to help you remove and discard any unnecessary, detrimental keys you may have on your key ring. Don't allow Satan to rob you of a success-ful journey by carrying any keys that are not beneficial to you. As you pray, choose to discard any unnecessary keys you have identified—leave them in the hands of the Father and ask Him to replace them with the true keys to success.

Father, I praise You and thank You, for Your divine power which has given me everything I need for life and godliness through my knowledge of You who called me by Your own glory and goodness (see 2 Peter 1:3). You have given me every key that I need to be victorious. Help me, Lord, to throw away any keys that I don't need. Help me to rely on You.

God, as one of Your chosen people, holy and dearly loved, help me to clothe myself with compassion, humility, gentleness and patience (see Colossians 3:12). Father, I really need the keys of patience and fortitude in my life. I am impatient with myself and with others. Fill me with a patient spirit as I give You my keys of impatience and weakness.

Almighty God, Your Word says that he who gets wisdom loves his own soul; and he who cherishes understanding prospers (see Proverbs 19:8). Father, I need *Your* wisdom, not the world's. I want understanding, not just knowledge. I want to understand more about You, Your Word and Your heart. Help me to obey You each day and to wisely use the keys I have learned about this week.

You have said that You give wisdom, Lord, and that from Your mouth come both knowledge and understanding (see Proverbs 2:6). Let me always listen to hear Your voice when You speak to my heart and when I read Your Word. Thank You for the wisdom You promise to give to those who seek it. How I pray that I will have the wisdom to treasure the keys to success that You have taught me this week. As I grow in knowledge and understanding of each, help me to fully incorporate them into my daily life and my Christian walk. And give me the courage to give You old keys that are not helpful to me.

DAY 7: *Reflections*

Keys can do so many different things. They can start an engine, open a door or lock a safe. In most cases keys are made to fit a specific keyhole; keys to one car won't work in another, for example. Usually, in a hotel or office, the manager and housekeepers have master keys they can use to open each individual room or office. However, on the inside of each room guests can choose to turn an internal security lock that will prevent or block the master key from working. Jesus is our master key, who can open every door, but He waits for permission from us to enter the door of our hearts, as well as the rooms of our hearts. Jesus won't force His way in; He waits for us to open the door. In Revelation 3:20, He says, "Here I am! I stand at the door and knock. If anyone hears my voice and opens the door, I will come in and eat with him, and he with me." Jesus is the single most important key to success that you can possess; He is the master key of life. He can open every door that we need opened, or He can lock doors we don't need to go through. He is the great shepherd who will lead us on the path to success when we allow Him to do so.

Have you opened the door of your heart to Him? It is so simple to do. Invite Him in today. If you have already asked Him into your heart, have you allowed Him to enter every room of your heart and life?

As you enter into prayer, begin by reviewing the memory verse for this week. Use the Scripture Memory Music CD and *Walking in the Word* to review each of the other verses that you have learned thus far. Frequent review will help you to fully establish each verse in your mind.

 Lord, You have told us that the thief comes to steal, kill and destroy; but that You come that we might have life, and that we might have abundant life (see John 10:10). Father, without You, nothing else matters. Your love and forgiveness for my sins overflow into my heart, cleanse me and give me hope and joy. Your promise of abundant life is an awesome promise that I humbly claim today. With You in my heart, I can have an abundant life filled with joy and peace.

My Redeemer, I know that it was not with perishable things such as silver and gold that I was redeemed from the empty way of life handed down to me from my forefathers, but with the precious blood of Christ, a lamb without blemish or defect (see 2 Peter 1:18-19).[1] Father, fill me with Your Spirit and help me to keep my whole heart open to You— cleanse every part.

Lord, You have shown me what is good and what You, Lord, require of me: to act justly, to love mercy and to walk humbly with You (see Micah 6:8).[2] Father, this week You have shown me the many good keys to success that will help me on this journey, and You have reminded me of the most important key—Jesus. Thank You, Lord, for I would be lost and helpless without You.

Notes
1. Beth Moore, *Praying God's Word* (Nashville, TN: Broadman and Holman, 2000), p. 145.
2. Ibid., p. 231.

GROUP PRAYER REQUESTS TODAY'S DATE:_____

NAME	REQUEST	RESULTS

THOUGHTS THAT BUILD SUCCESS

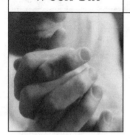

Week Six

Is your mind programmed for success? Or do you play destructive, self-defeating tapes in your head? The language of success must be programmed into our minds, and the negative tapes must be deleted. In this week's study we will examine some common thoughts that will either hinder or help us succeed.

DAY 1: *Confidence*

Our perspective—our viewpoint on life—affects our potential for success. A story from the book of Numbers demonstrates how differently people can view the same situation. Do you have confidence that God is working through you?

In Numbers 13:1-3,17—14:10, Moses sent leaders from each tribe to investigate the Promised Land of Canaan.

➤ How would you describe the response and perspective of Joshua and Caleb?

➤ How would you describe the response and perspective of the other spies?

➤ Have you encountered any giants or powerful enemies since you started First Place? Describe them.

➤ When you encounter your giants, what is your response?

- ☐ To want to give in to fear like the other spies
- ☐ To boldly step out in faith like Joshua and Caleb

Our perspective will make a difference in how we view the challenges of life. When we walk close to God, the giants cannot get near enough to overpower us. Determine to have confidence, believing that God is on your side and will help you win. Praise Him for the victories yet to come.

Begin learning this week's memory verse—approach the learning process with confidence that you can learn to memorize Scripture. Play the Scripture Memory Music CD and use *Walking in the Word* to help you. Review daily.

Heavenly Father, help me to remember that with You on my side, I can win the battles against the giants in my life.

O Lord, give me Your confidence as I choose to boldly step out in faith when I face difficulties or enter into unknown territory.

DAY 2: *Wise Choices*

While Cindy was married, she became furious with her husband when he ordered for her in a restaurant. He thought his selection would be a healthier choice than anything Cindy might order. Cindy refused to eat it. She didn't want to be told what to do. Later, she realized that although her husband may have overstepped his boundaries, he was trying to help her. Cindy could have responded by expressing appreciation for her husband's desire to help her and by choosing wisely. A rebellious spirit caused her to miss a blessing!

⤳ According to James 3:13,17-18, what are the qualities of someone who makes wise choices?

⤳ List one or more of these qualities that would help you make healthy lifestyle choices.

⤳ Read the following stories of encounters with Jesus. Check the kind of response each person made.

	Wise choice	Unwise choice
Matthew 4:18-22	☐	☐
Matthew 9:9	☐	☐
Matthew 19:16-22	☐	☐
Matthew 26:7	☐	☐
Mark 6:1-5	☐	☐

When God created us He gave us the ability to choose. We can choose His way or our own way. First Place is dedicated to helping us make wise lifestyle choices, mentally, emotionally, spiritually and physically.

⤳ Evaluate the choices you've made this past week in regard to the nine First Place commitments.

	Wise choices	Unwise choices
Attendance	☐	☐
Prayer	☐	☐
Scripture reading	☐	☐
Memory verse	☐	☐
Bible study	☐	☐
Live-It plan	☐	☐
Commitment Records	☐	☐
Encouragement	☐	☐
Exercise	☐	☐

Praise God for any wise responses that you marked. Remember that His power allows you to make wise choices. Decide to wisely consider the many choices you will need to make this week. Wisely choose how you will spend your time. Consider including time to do the following:

- Encourage a fellow group member with a note or phone call.
- Seek the Lord early each day through prayer, Bible study and Scripture reading.
- Start a new exercise to add variety to current activities.
- Serve someone in need—take a meal to an elderly neighbor or volunteer to help at your church.
- Other:_____

Thank You, Lord, for helping me to make wise choices regarding my nine First Place commitments. Help me when I falter in my choices.

Father, help me to seek Your will in all my choices.

DAY 3: *A Hopeful Heart and Healthy Self-Esteem*

First, we must realize that thoughts of hopelessness lead us into despair, but thoughts of *hopefulness* lead us to glad anticipation of a victorious future.

➤ According to Romans 15:12-13, what must we do in order to experience an overflow of hope?

➤ What will happen as we put our trust in the God of hope?

Paul knew firsthand that relying on his own strength would not suffice. In 2 Corinthians 1:8-11, he praised God for reminding him that his sufferings "happened that we might not rely on ourselves but on God." Hope springs from trusting God to gain the victory, rather than trying to win the battles by our own strength.

>> In what areas of your life are you feeling hopeless?

>> In what areas are you feeling hopeful?

Read the testimonies in the First Place newsletter and in the book *Choosing to Change* by Carole Lewis, First Place national director. Testimonies of those who have succeeded encourage us to keep pursuing our goals.

If you are hindered by thoughts of hopelessness, pray as Paul did in Ephesians 1:18-19. Pray that your eyes will be opened and you will be able to see and "know the hope to which he has called you, the riches of his glorious inheritance in the saints, and his incomparably great power for us who believe."

We must also realize that having healthy self-esteem greatly influences our potential to experience success. Our self-esteem is greatly influenced by what we allow into our minds. Therefore, it is important to consider this question: Do you listen to and believe the negative messages others install in your brain? These messages need to be filtered by God's virus-protection program! God's Word assures us that everyone who accepts Him is a new creation (see 2 Corinthians 5:17). We do not have to be haunted by replays of past failures or current shortcomings. We do not have to be influenced by the negative words of others. We can evaluate what is said and then act on any truths that need to be addressed or erase any messages that are not true. We must recognize that we are of great worth to our Lord.

➣ What assurance of your value to God is found in Matthew 6:26?

➣ How will believing you are of infinite worth to the Lord help you succeed in the First Place program?

Although we come to Christ just as we are, He loves us too much to let us stay that way. He wants the best for us and knows that through His power all things are possible. After Cindy began to deal with her low self-esteem, she had to reprogram her mind with the truth of who she was in Christ, knowing that He could and would continue to do His mighty work in her. He will do the same for you. He is able!

➣ Write the words from Deuteronomy 7:6-9 that indicate your value and worth to God.

Do not allow anyone to program your mind with thoughts that will hinder you. As a child of the King, believe that you are a new creation—the old things have passed away!

 Write or say a prayer of thanksgiving to the One who loved you so much that He was willing to die in your place.

DAY 4: *Availability and Persistence*

Have you ever thought, *I am too old and too set in my ways to accomplish great things for God,* or *I am too young—I don't know enough about life or about the Bible—how can God use someone like me?*

Cindy was asked to teach a women's Sunday School class several years ago. She felt too young spiritually and was overwhelmed by a sense of inadequacy. She eventually accepted the position, believing God had called her to this task and that He would equip her to do it.

❧ After reading the following Scriptures, write the age (or age group) of the person involved and what he or she accomplished for God:

	Age	Accomplishment
2 Kings 5:2-4,14		
2 Kings 22:1-2		
Luke 1:5-15,18,23-25		
John 6:9-13		
Hebrews 11:11-12		

❧ In 1 Timothy 4:12-16, what did Paul say about how age affects our ability to serve God?

❧ In what ways have you used your physical or spiritual age or experience as an excuse to keep from obeying God's directions to you?

When we are available, God uses us. Perhaps you are familiar with the story of a crippled English lad who wrote Scripture verses and tossed them out his upstairs window. Passersby read this little lad's messages, and through them many were touched by the Spirit. Whatever your age—physically or spiritually—God can do mighty things through you.

Thank God for every precious day of life that He gives. If you believe it is too late for you or that you are too young, "Be transformed by the renewing of your mind" (Romans 12:2). Let Psalm 148:7,12-13 be your song of praise today: "Praise the LORD . . . young men and maidens, old men and children. Let them praise the name of the LORD, for his name alone is exalted; his splendor is above the earth and the heavens." Tell God you are available to Him, to be used according to His plan.

In addition to instructing us to make ourselves available to God, the Bible also urges us to be persistent, to continue on even when we stumble and fall. Three steps forward and one step back still put us two steps ahead! Five pounds lost and two pounds gained still result in a net loss of three pounds! Even if you lose two and gain five, if you will stop, evaluate, re-commit and persevere, you will eventually make your goal! Be persistent, no matter what! This truth applies to other goals as well, not just weight-management goals.

➳ According to Hebrews 10:36, what do we receive if we persevere?

The writer of Hebrews urged us to keep on in our faith. We need to practice what we have learned even though those around us are living a different lifestyle. Many people outside your First Place group lead un-healthy lifestyles. When you are with them, focus on your new lifestyle. Persisting in the nine commitments will give you the fulfillment of the promise of a healthy lifestyle.

➳ After reading Colossians 1:21-24, complete the following sentence:

If you continue in your faith, Christ will present you_____

_____in His sight.

Do you need to make a deeper commitment to keeping the Com-mitment Record, your exercise routine, drinking eight glasses of water or writing in your prayer journal?

✎ List those activities to which you need to recommit.

James 1:4 says that perseverance leads to maturity. Continue on today to learn your memory verse and to pursue your goals with renewed dedication.

 Thank You, Father, that You never give up on me! Please give me strength and the mind-set to be persistent for Your glory.

DAY 5: *Optimism*

When you look at a water glass with some water in it, do you think of it as half empty or half full? An optimistic spirit looks on the bright side, expecting the best, because God is able! The I-can mind-set finds strength in God rather than self.

✎ What did God tell Moses in Exodus 3:10?

✎ What were the I-can't thoughts in Moses' reply in Exodus 3:11,13 and 4:1,10?

✎ What was God's response to Moses' negative attitude in Exodus 4:14?

Moses did not have the confidence to do what God asked. God knew Moses' apprehensions and inadequacies, but God also knew that Moses plus God equaled sufficiency!

➤ According to 4:14-17, what was God's solution to Moses' lack of faith?

Just as God sent Aaron to help Moses, we can have confidence that God will use First Place leaders and group members, and perhaps others, to help us believe in ourselves so that we do what is necessary to accomplish our goals.

➤ What are some I-can't thoughts that are temporarily hindering you?

➤ Now write Philippians 4:13 and then read each of your I-can't thoughts followed by Philippians 4:13.

 Father God, please help me develop an I-can-with-God's-help mind-set that will enable me to move forward on the path with thoughts that build success in my life.

DAY 6: *Reflections*

This week's study focused on thoughts. The information that our minds receive becomes the basis for our thoughts. Our brains store information much like the hard drive on a computer. Therefore, just as with a computer, it is crucial to install the right kind of information in our minds. The familiar "garbage in—garbage out" also applies to our minds. We must be compelled to consider what we put into our minds if we want to produce thoughts and attitudes that will be productive and positive. Our success or failure can easily be determined by what and how we think. Garbage thoughts (*I can't do this; I give up; This is just too hard; What's the point; I will never succeed;* etc.) tend to produce garbage results and ultimately lead to failure. In contrast, valuable thoughts (*Nothing is impossible with God's help; I can do this; I can learn to lead a more disciplined life; I will reach the goals God has planned for me; I can overcome temptation;* etc.) will ultimately lead to success.

As we fill our minds and hearts with God's Word, we can replace the garbage with treasure. Review your memory verse and faithfully study God's Word so that your mind and heart can be filled with His power and with His Word—the best source for thoughts that build success!

Now allow the following Scripture prayers to usher you into the presence of almighty God, your loving heavenly Father who eagerly awaits fellowship with you.

Father, Your Word exhorts me to set my mind on things above, not on earthly things (see Colossians 3:2). This can be such a battle, Lord! Please help me every single day to set my mind on You.[1] Fill my mind with great treasures; help me to get rid of the garbage that is already in my mind. I realize that I must do my part, but I am depending on You for strength and power to do it.

Lord, You have said that Your thoughts are not like my thoughts, and Your ways are not like my ways. Your Word tells me that just as the heavens are higher than the earth, so are Your ways higher than my ways and Your thoughts are higher than mine (see Isaiah 55:8-9). Oh, Lord, I want and need to think more like You do, because without Your influence my thoughts and my ways so easily sabotage and defeat me. Let my thoughts be fashioned by the power of Your Word, Your love and Your grace. Let my thoughts and my ways come from the confident hope and magnificent power of Your Spirit in me.

Lord, Your Word tells me that You are the one who forms the mountains and creates the wind and that You reveal Your thoughts to humans. You turn the dawn to darkness and tread the high places of the earth; Lord God Almighty is Your name (see Amos 4:13). Father, it is beyond the comprehension of my finite, human mind that You, the God who created this world and everything in it, would reveal Your thoughts to us—to me! Help my heart to listen so that I will hear You when You speak, when You reveal Your thoughts to me as I pray and study Your Word. May Your thoughts and Your Word form thoughts in my mind that build success in my life—but only success in the plans and goals You desire for me.

DAY 7: *Reflections*

As you conclude this week's study on "Thoughts That Build Success," review the instructions in Philippians 4:7-8: "The peace of God, which transcends all understanding, will guard your hearts and your minds in Christ Jesus. Finally, brothers, whatever is true, whatever is noble, whatever is right, whatever is pure, whatever is lovely, whatever is admirable—if anything is excellent or praiseworthy—think about such things."

Virtually everything we see, hear, touch and experience can be a source from which our thoughts are formed. We must be prudent about the many things that can influence our minds: television programs, movies, books, radio programs, music, speakers, magazines and more.

Consider taking a little time today to make a mental or perhaps written list of examples of the kinds of things we are encouraged to think about in this passage from Philippians. Sources include, but are not limited to, the Bible, Christian music, poetry, literature, art, God's creation, God Himself—His character, His promises, His deeds, personal testimonies of Christians, biographies and autobiographies of great men and women of God.

Father God, I praise You for the truth You have given in Romans 8:31: "If God is for us, who can be against us?" Lord, this is a powerful thought for me to grasp: You are on my side, and no one can stand against You! Thank You, Lord.

Sweet Lord, it is good to praise You and make music to Your name, O Most High. It is wonderful to proclaim Your love in the morning when I get up and Your faithfulness at night before I fall asleep—I do so with music and singing in my heart. For You make me glad by Your deeds, O Lord; I sing for joy at the works of Your hands. How great are Your works, O Lord, and how profound are Your thoughts (see Psalm 92:1-5). Father, it is true—when I spend time with You and I study Your Word and allow You to fill my mind and soul, then my thoughts and my heart are changed. You fill me with peace, joy and hope. Oh, how the thought floods over my soul, Lord, when I realize from this verse I am one of the works of Your mighty hand. Please let this thought stay with me, Lord. Let it compel me to think better of myself and to take better care of myself through understanding that I am valuable to You and also to follow the commitments in First Place.

Heavenly Father, Your Word tells me that You are able to do immeasurably more than all I could ask or even begin to imagine, according to Your power at work within me, to You be all the glory (see Ephesians 3:20-21). I praise You and thank You, Lord, that You are fully able to help me guard my thoughts. Teach me to ask for things that would please You, Father. Fill me with Your Spirit and power, which will enable me to follow through with the commitments.

Note
1. Beth Moore, *Praying God's Word* (Nashville, TN: Broadman and Holman, 2000), p. 145.

GROUP PRAYER REQUESTS   TODAY'S DATE:_____

NAME	REQUEST	RESULTS

OVERCOMING LEADS TO SUCCESS

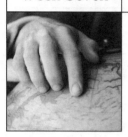

MEMORY VERSE

Everyone born of God overcomes the world. This is the victory that has overcome the world, even our faith. Who is it that overcomes the world? Only he who believes that Jesus is the Son of God.

1 John 5:4-5

When Cindy began First Place, she had to overcome the effects of low self-esteem that contributed to her weight problem. Every human being faces obstacles and challenges in life. Perhaps you are currently experiencing a turbulent time. Will you be one who overcomes? In order to succeed, you must choose to confront the troubles, obstacles and challenges of your life with faith in God to provide the victory (see Psalm 139:23-24).

DAY 1: *Overcoming Habits*

Cindy had the habit of using the elevator at work, although her office was on the second floor. One day a coworker challenged her to climb the stairs instead. She began to use the stairs at least once a day. Gradually, it became a habit. Comfortable ways of doing things may keep you from being successful. Through First Place and God's Word, look at habits that may not be in your best interest.

➤ According to Colossians 2:6-8, what is the result of following human traditions, or habits, and principles?

➤ Whose ways should we follow?

Faith that overcomes our habits discovers the power to do so through the following three-point path to victory:

1. Seek God's power daily through prayer.
2. Seek God's direction through the study of His Word as you endeavor to form new habits.
3. Seek help from others by being accountable to First Place members or to a fellow believer.

God's children must think and behave differently from worldly men and women.

≫ Do you have some habits that need to change?

☐ Yes   ☐ No

≫ Are you willing to seek God's power and guidance to change?

☐ Yes   ☐ No

≫ How are you seeking help from others?

≫ List one or two good habits that you want to develop.

Habits are built slowly over time by repeating certain behaviors. New habits are built the same way—day by day, action by action. Pray about your responses to today's questions and ask God to reveal habits you need to change. Continue to develop the habit of Scripture memory. Begin learning this week's verse and spend a few minutes reviewing and quoting the memory verses you have learned in the previous weeks.

Almighty God, thank You that I do not need to make these changes of habit alone because You have overcome the world. In times of discouragement, O Lord, remind me that I can have a fresh start in You and that You will grant me the desires of my heart to live a healthy, balanced life.

DAY 2: *Overcoming Mistakes; False Expectations*

All of us learn by trial and error—it is part of life's learning process. However, some mistakes should never happen and can be avoided altogether if we apply godly wisdom and guidance to our lives. Sometimes we make mistakes that lead us to sin. Failing to overcome mistakes and sin can hinder our success. Similarly, sometimes we have wrong expectations that can interfere with our ability to succeed. When we presume to know how God should work in our lives, we need to ask for God's help. Today's lesson will explore the source of power that will enable us to overcome mistakes and sin, as well as false expectations.

The story of David and Bathsheba is recorded in 2 Samuel 11. Read the story and then answer the following:

➤ Could David have avoided his mistakes that led to sin?

☐ Yes   ☐ No

➤ Can we avoid mistakes that lead to sin in our lives?

☐ Yes   ☐ No

David made the mistake of not being where he should have been; he stayed home in the spring, the time when kings went off to war (see 2 Samuel 11:1). This was David's first mistake, and it led to all the others. His second mistake was to watch Bathsheba as she bathed. When he realized that a woman was bathing, he should have turned his eyes away. Instead, David kept looking; he looked long enough to notice that Bathsheba was beautiful. His next mistake was to send messengers to bring her to him. The situation continued to worsen as David's mistakes led to sin. Yes, David could have avoided his mistakes and his sin. Further, if he had confessed his sin and asked for forgiveness rather than trying to cover it up, David could have avoided compounding his sin.

In 2 Samuel 12:1-13, the prophet Nathan rebuked David for his sin. Read Psalm 51. Although David and others suffered the consequences of his mistakes and sins, overcoming them through true confession and repentance led David to a changed heart, a heart cleansed and restored to God.

≫ Place a check beside the actions David called on God to perform.

☐ Cleanse   ☐ Blot out transgressions

☐ Renew a steadfast spirit   ☐ Wash away all iniquity

☐ Take the Holy Spirit   ☐ Cast away from God's presence
  from him

≫ Do you need God to restore the joy of your salvation today?

≫ After reading 1 John 1:9, fill in the blanks.

If we confess our_____, He is_____

and just and will_____us our sins and purify us

from all_____.

John provided the following three-point process for overcoming the effects of our sin:

1. Conviction and awareness of sin

2. Confession of sin

3. Repentance and cleansing from sin

Relying on God as our help, we can avoid mistakes that lead to sin. His power can help us to do our part, which includes avoiding being in the wrong place at the wrong time, turning our eyes away from temptation and making right choices. When you do make a mistake that leads to sin, ask for God's forgiveness and grace.

To overcome mistakes and sins, we need to allow God to cleanse us and then to begin anew. A heart that is cleansed from sin has renewed strength, hope and power to live for the Lord. Ask God to "renew a steadfast spirit" within you today (see Psalm 51:10).

Overcoming both mistakes and false expectations can help us on our journey to success. Expectations should be realistic. For example, what are your expectations about the First Place program? Do you have realistic expectations about the amount of weight that you should be able to lose in a session? Realistic expectations challenge us; unrealistic expectations will discourage us. Ultimately, our hope for success should be placed in Jesus Christ. He is our model and power source for overcoming the obstacles we face.

Consider Matthew 11:1-10. John the Baptist had spent his life preparing for and expecting the Messiah. He wanted to be sure his expectations were being fulfilled in Jesus.

➤ What did Jesus say was the proof of His identity? Check all that apply.

☐ He wore fine clothes. ☐ He lived in a palace.
☐ The blind could see. ☐ The dead were raised to life.
☐ The lame could walk. ☐ He prophesied.
☐ The deaf could hear. ☐ Good news was preached to
☐ Lepers were cured. the poor.

Jesus knew the people were expecting another kind of Messiah. Like the people of Jesus' day, we may be disappointed if we expect the Christian life to be a life of comfort, wealth and continuous emotional highs.

➤ What unrealistic expectations about being a Christian have you had?

➤ Do you have faith that God by His mighty power will help you reach your goals and dreams?

☐ Yes ☐ No

➤ Are you confident that Jesus is the One who can save and deliver you?

☐ Yes ☐ No

➤ Do you have realistic weight-loss goals that are in line with God's plans for you?

☐ Yes   ☐ No

➤ Consider your expectations for yourself and others. Are they realistic? Are they healthy and wise?

Just as we have certain expectations of Jesus, He has expectations of us. We can expect the Christian life to produce Christlike character, faith that endures the hard tests of time and power to overcome temptations. These are realistic expectations!

Holy God, search my heart and show me what expectations You have for me.

Help me, Lord, to make right choices and avoid mistakes that lead to sin.

DAY 3: Overcoming Willfulness

How do you respond to instruction? Do you prefer to set your own rules and be your own boss? A degree of independence is healthy; but carried to an extreme, it may result in a willful, disobedient and rebellious response to God's authority. Evaluate how you react to God's sovereignty in your life.

➤ Describe the heart attitude of the people in Deuteronomy 31:27.

➤ Do you struggle with rebellion in regard to any of the nine First Place commitments? Check those that are a problem for you.

□ Attendance   □ Memory verse   □ Commitment Record
□ Prayer   □ Bible study   □ Encouragement
□ Scripture reading □ Live-It plan   □ Exercise

In your prayer journal, record any of the commitments that you checked, as well as anything else you feel rebellious about. Pray about these during the remainder of this week and ask God to help you overcome this heart attitude.

➤ After reading 1 Samuel 15:22-23, fill in the blanks.

Samuel compared_____to divination and _____to the evil of idolatry.

➤ What does this passage tell you about the seriousness of the sins of rebellion and arrogance?

➤ In your own words, define a willful person.

➤ Which of the following words describe your response to God's rightful authority in your life? Check all that apply.

□ Rebelliousness   □ Willfulness
□ Attentiveness   □ Obedience
□ Stubbornness   □ Rejection

➤ Read Psalm 119:10-16 to discover the actions of an obedient heart. List the corresponding action beside each verse.

• Verse 10

• Verse 11

- Verse 12

- Verse 13

- Verse 14

- Verse 15

- Verse 16

As you pray today, share with God the desire of your heart.

 Father, I ask forgiveness for the willfulness I have displayed in the past. I commit to becoming a more obedient child of Yours, loving Father. I commit to hiding Your Word in my heart and ask that You would give me the power to overcome.

DAY 4: *Overcoming Limitations*

What kinds of things limit you? Education? Temperament? Physical condition? Financial status? Adverse circumstances? God's Word assures us that we can overcome limitations that would defeat His purposes for our lives. As you study, consider any limitations you may be facing. Surrender yourself and your limitations to the Lord, allowing Him to move you above and beyond those limitations.

➺ According to Acts 4:1-2,8-13, what limitations did Peter and John have?

➺ What was the reaction of the people?

≫ What did the people notice?

≫ Read the following Scripture passages and match them with the limitations that were overcome:

_____ Genesis 21:9-20   a. Adverse circumstances

_____ 1 Kings 17:1-4,7-16   b. Temperament

_____ 2 Kings 4:1-7   c. Physical condition

_____ Matthew 15:32-39   d. Limited resources

_____ Luke 5:17-26   e. Financial needs

≫ Describe an occasion when you have experienced God's help in overcoming limitations.

≫ With regard to your potential success in First Place, what limitations do you need to deal with?

≫ Do you need an extra measure of faith to overcome these limitations? The last phrase of Acts 4:13 reveals the secret to having faith that overcomes. What is the secret?

Father God, please give me courage to face my limitations. I know that my faith and trust in You will empower me to overcome them.

DAY 5: Overcoming Temptations and Doubts

Temptations and doubts of one kind or another plague everyone. For anyone dealing with weight management and attempting to make healthy lifestyle choices, temptation and doubt can be major problems to overcome. Our level of success in life, as well as in First Place, will definitely be measured by how we cope with doubts and how well we handle the many temptations we encounter each day.

Hebrews 2:18 tells us that Jesus understands temptation.

➤ What is Jesus able to do for those who are tempted?

➤ What are the two steps outlined in James 4:7 that will help us overcome temptation?

➤ What is the end result of these steps?

➤ According to Luke 22:31-32, Jesus warned Simon Peter that his faith was about to be tested. What did Jesus assure Simon He had done for him, and why?

➤ According to Luke 22:34, what did Jesus know about how Simon Peter would respond to being sifted by Satan?

Jesus told Simon Peter to strengthen his brothers after his temptation experience was over. Consider how Jesus can use your battles with temptation to strengthen other members of your First Place group. We can learn and grow through the failures and successes of others.

When you are tempted, remember that you have a High Priest, Jesus Christ Himself, who was tempted as you are and yet did not sin (see Hebrews 4:15-16). Because He understands your temptations, He has provided a power source to help you resist them. Call on your power source, the Holy Spirit, today. He will help you overcome the temptations and lead you to success!

If you had asked Cindy if she would lose 100 pounds in First Place, she would have replied, "I doubt it." Do you doubt that you will ever reach your First Place goals? Do you require tangible evidence before believing? Faith in God's power at work in your life can dispel your doubts and disbelief.

➣ In Matthew 17:15-20, how much faith did Jesus say we need in order to accomplish what seems to be impossible?

➣ After reading Hebrews 11:1, use your own words to describe what faith is.

Have you ever thought, *I can never drink eight or more glasses of water every day; I will never like exercise; I can't crowd one more thing into my life; I can't memorize Scripture?* Many First Place members have testified to having had such thoughts. But when their bodies experienced the benefits of a healthy lifestyle, they were encouraged to reach goals they had felt were unreachable.

If you are having trouble believing you can attain your goals, ask your First Place group members how they deal with their doubts about keeping the commitments or staying on the path to success. Someone else's testimony can help lead you down the pathway to success in overcoming doubt.

Considering Mark 9:17-24, what unbelief would you like God's help with today?

Heavenly Father, help me overcome my doubts and disbelief. I ask You to increase my faith so that I can also say, "I do believe; help me overcome my unbelief" (see Mark 9:24).

DAY 6: *Reflections*

The theme of this week's study is overcoming. The memory verse taught us that our faith is the victory that overcomes the world. As we overcome the things that hinder us, we are taking the steps that lead us to success in accomplishing our goals and dreams; these steps also lead us to success in building a stronger faith and relationship in our walk with God. So what is faith? It begins with being born of God—believing in Him and in His Son, Jesus. Faith involves our complete dependence on God; it is reflected in a heart that is willing to trust and obey.

As you begin your prayer time today, reflect again on the following passage from Luke, which was discussed on Day 5: "The apostles said to the Lord, 'Increase our faith!' He replied, 'If you have faith as small as a mustard seed, you can say to this mulberry tree, "Be uprooted and planted in the sea," and it will obey you'" (Luke 17:5-6). Praise God that even faith as small as a mustard seed is enough faith to overcome and lead you to success. Ask the Lord to let your heart echo the request: *Increase my faith*.

Heavenly Father, Your Word teaches me that showing love for You means obeying Your commands. You say that Your commands are not burdensome, because everyone born of God overcomes the world. Only those who believe that Jesus is the Son of God overcome the world (see 1 John 5:3-5). Lord, I believe in You and Your Son, Jesus. Lord, help me to obey You each day and to trust You more. Help me to claim the victory You have won for me. I am an overcomer through You!

Father, You have called us Your dear children, and You have said that we are from You and have overcome the evil one because the One who is in us is greater than the one who is in the world (see 1 John 4:4). Father, Your power in me is my strength to overcome; without You I am powerless.

Lord, Your Word says that some trust in chariots and some in horses, but we trust in the name of the LORD our God. They are brought to their knees and fall, but we rise up and stand firm (see Psalm 20:7-8). My faith is in You, Lord, not in my possessions, strength or money. I will overcome by my faith and trust in You. Increase my faith, Lord.

DAY 7: *Reflections*

Those who face the challenge to overcome need hope to keep going while they wait on God's timing. The victory belongs to those who place their hopes and dreams in God through faith. Despite the odds against you, success can be yours if you refuse to give up hope. God is able to do mighty things by His awesome power. His promises are true. Keep your faith and trust in Him alive and growing. Depend on Him to help you overcome your habits, mistakes, sins, false expectations, willfulness, rebellion, limitations, temptations and doubts—just as Abraham and many other saints of old did.

The book of Romans records the account of Abraham's faith and hope in God.

Against all hope, Abraham in hope believed and so became the father of many nations, just as it had been said to him, "So shall your offspring be." Without weakening in his faith, he faced the fact that his body was as good as dead—since he was about a hundred years old—and that Sarah's womb was also dead. Yet he did not waver through unbelief regarding the promise of God, but was strengthened in his faith and gave glory to God, being fully persuaded that God had power to do what he had promised (Romans 4:18-21).

Ponder two questions as you prepare for prayer: Are you hoping against all hope, believing by faith that He is able to keep His promises regarding you? Are you fully persuaded that He has the power to do what He has promised in your life? Use the following Scripture prayers to ask God to help you remain faithful to Him and to the First Place commitments. Thank Him for the reason for your hope—Jesus, the object of your faith.

Lord, Your Word says that faith is being sure of what we hope for and certain of what we do not see (see Hebrews 11:1). My confidence is in You, Lord. I believe with all my heart that You will help my faith grow. I have faith that You will help me overcome obstacles and that the things I hope for, but can't see just yet, will come about in Your perfect timing.

Father God, I know that You have told me these things, so that in You I can have peace. You said that we would have trouble in this world. We will experience obstacles to overcome, but You have told me to take heart, to have hope, because You have overcome the world (see John 16:33).

Lord Most High, I pray that the eyes of my heart may be enlightened so that I may know the hope to which You have called me, the riches of Your glorious inheritance in the saints and Your incomparably great power for all of us who believe (see Ephesians 1:19). Let me steadfastly put my hope and faith in You to help me overcome the problems and challenges in my life with Your great power, believing that overcoming leads to the success of Your plans and visions for my life.

You, O Lord, are my God of hope. Fill me with all joy and peace as I trust in You so that I may overflow with hope by the power of the Holy Spirit (see Romans 15:13). Father, thank You for Your presence and hope. I trust my life to You. By Your power, lead me on the pathway to success and fill me with overflowing hope and faith that overcomes.

GROUP PRAYER REQUESTS   TODAY'S DATE:_____

NAME	REQUEST	RESULTS

STAYING ON TRACK TO SUCCESS

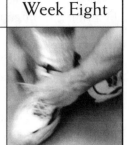

MEMORY VERSE

Whether you turn to the right or to the left,
your ears will hear a voice behind you, saying,
"This is the way; walk in it."
Isaiah 30:21

As you progress on your pathway to success, you may discover the road has few travelers, for many who begin do not stay on course. Even if the road is lonely and you encounter many billboards tempting you away, beware—do not let them distract and sidetrack you along the way. The journey may be difficult and strenuous at times, but for those who stay on track there will be great rewards.

DAY 1: *Stop Signs*

What do you do when you come to a stop sign? Are you cautious as you approach the intersection? Do you come to a complete stop? Do you look in all directions before you proceed? Stop signs and traffic lights offer safety and protection as you travel. Today, we will study some biblical stop signs and traffic lights on the pathway to success.

➤ After reading Job 37:14, complete the following:

Like Job, we need to_____and_____
the wonders of God.

➤ In Acts 1:1-4, what stop sign did the disciples receive from Jesus and why did He give it?

When good things have happened, we often want to rush on to the next challenge. Waiting for direction for the future requires patience and maturity. The stop signs of life have a purpose. Don't miss God's purposes by rushing through them or only slowing down. Come to a complete stop—until God directs you to move.

At times, God asks us to come to a complete stop and evaluate our lives to consider where we are and where we are going. Sometimes our lives come to a screeching halt, forcing us to come face-to-face with the realities of life. Painful realities might include caring for an aging parent, facing cancer or standing at the graveside of a loved one. Happier realities also cause us to stop and evaluate our lives: graduations, job promotions, the birth of a child, a new home.

When you joined First Place, did you sense or experience an abrupt stop sign when you first weighed in? Think about how God advised you to proceed on your journey toward a healthy lifestyle.

➤ How have the stop signs in your life been God's protection for you as you traveled the pathway to success?

➤ What was one specific stop sign that had a definite purpose in your life?

Genesis 19 tells the story of the destruction of the cities of Sodom and Gomorrah. Read Genesis 19:12-17. What instructions did the angels give to Lot and his family?

➤ What did the angels tell them *not* to do (v. 17)?

≫ What happened to Lot's wife (v. 26)?

≫ What lesson do you learn from Lot's wife's mistake?

Be careful not to create a stop sign where God does not want you to stop. Stopping in the wrong place at the wrong time can easily lead us into trouble or cause us to turn in a wrong direction. Be alert to God's instructions in order to stay on track to success, stopping only where He instructs.

≫ According to Psalm 46:10, what is the purpose of being still?

Is it hard for you to find time to be still? An ordinary day in Cindy's life always seemed so busy. Her time was consumed with work, caring for her children, helping with homework, racing from one after-school activity to another, attending soccer practice and games, grocery shopping, cooking and tending to household chores; she had to fit in attendance at church, choir rehearsal, First Place and family gatherings. The word "busy" aptly described her life. Then one day on a bulletin board at her office she read a phrase that stopped her cold: "Beware of the barrenness of a busy life!" Cindy realized that she needed to find a way to slow down, to stop and take time each day to be still before the Lord.

If we fail to observe the stop signs, we are in danger of forgetting God. We can easily forget He is in charge and in control of our future. We can get off track without the instructions and guidance He gives when we spend time with Him.

Take time from the activities of your busy day to stop and savor time in the Father's presence. Take time to begin learning the memory verse for this week; then listen to the verse on the Scripture Memory Music CD and keep *Walking in the Word* with you for quick review when you are waiting at traffic lights.

 Heavenly Father, help me to learn to stop and be still before You so that I can know You better. Guide me in finding those quiet times and places when I can listen to You.

Help me, Lord, to recognize Your stop signs and obey them.

DAY 2: *Construction Ahead—Detours and Distractions*

Have you heard the expression "Be patient; God isn't through with me yet"? "Construction Ahead" signs remind us that work is in progress; God is not through with us. Construction will help prepare us for the work God wants to do in us and through us.

➺ Consider 1 Peter 2:5; why is God building spiritual houses out of us as His living stones?

➺ According to Philippians 1:6, how long will God's good work in us be under construction?

➺ According to 2 Corinthians 9:8, what does God give us to make us abound in every good work?

Just as individuals must cooperate with God, the Church is built up when individuals cooperate with the Master Builder.

➤ According to Ephesians 4:16, what is required of each member of the Church body in order for it to grow?

When you joined First Place, God began a mighty construction project in you. Consider the following questions:

➤ Are you cooperating with the Master Builder and Designer?

☐ Yes   ☐ No

➤ Are you allowing Him to work on His schedule?

☐ Yes   ☐ No

➤ Have you caused some unnecessary delays?

☐ Yes   ☐ No

Pray for patience with yourself and others as God does His construction work. Be a faithful and diligent worker when God gives you a task. Record in your prayer journal or in the margin ways you can be a more faithful part of your church and your First Place group.

Are you easily distracted from your goal? Do you ever take a wrong turn or even an exit? We all have strayed off course at one time or another. When we allow the flesh to be in charge rather than the Holy Spirit, we get off track and succumb to the many alluring distractions and tempting detours this world has to offer. Be sensitive to God's direction and get back on track as soon as possible!

➤ According to Psalm 119:35,133, how will following God's path and directions for you keep you from taking unnecessary detours and U-turns?

➻ In Matthew 26:41, what strategy did Jesus encourage the disciples to use to avoid temptation?

➻ How well do you utilize prayer when faced with temptations? Check one.

☐ Very little   ☐ Often
☐ Some of the time   ☐ All of the time

➻ What distracts or tempts you to get off track?

➻ According to 1 Corinthians 10:13, what does God promise to do for us when we face temptations?

When you are tempted to get off the right pathway, remember that God has provided a way of escape for you. Sometimes God provides a detour around the distractions and temptations, but often He expects us to face temptations squarely and with His help come out victorious on the other side.

The story of Jonah is a classic example of a man who took an unnecessary detour and had to make a U-turn in order to get back on the path God had ordained for him. God told Jonah to go to the city of Nineveh to preach to the people, but Jonah ran away from the Lord's appointed path. When he came to his senses, Jonah cried out to God for help and grace. God gave him a second chance to be obedient. Jonah preached in Nineveh, and the people repented of their sins because Jonah had obeyed God.

Are you steadfastly keeping to your appointed path in regard to the First Place program? If not, ask God for forgiveness and grace; then start again. Faithfully follow God's road. He will bless your obedience.

Father God, thank You that You continue to do Your good work in me. Help me avoid the detours that would distract me from the path You have planned for me.

Lord, remind me that You will provide a way of escape when I am tempted to follow a detour.

Day 3: *Rest Stops and Warning Signs*

When Cindy entered First Place, she wanted to lose weight immediately. It seemed so unfair when someone else lost weight faster than she did. Each of us progresses along the pathway to success at an individual pace. Although we may want to reach our destination quickly, God has placed rest stops along the way. What do you think are the purposes of rest stops? Do you need occasional rest stops on your journey?

➣ According to Jeremiah 6:16, how do you find rest for your soul?

Ask where the _____ is and

_____ in it.

➣ Record your impressions about the rest stops indicated in each of the following Scripture passages:

- Psalm 37:7-8

- Psalm 62:5-6

- James 5:7-8

Rest stops are intended to remind us of God's presence and help us experience His peace. They are not intended as a rest stop from healthy living.

➣ Where are you in your pilgrimage in the First Place program? Check one.

☐ Lagging behind
☐ Progressing on schedule
☐ Hurrying impatiently

Ask yourself how being in too big a hurry affects all areas of your life, not just First Place. Take time to record in your journal what God reveals to you, and share with the class the insights you gleaned.

God sets a different course for each of us. When you follow the First Place program, be assured that the pace at which you progress is the speed that is designed for you. Pay attention to the rest stops God provides along the way. Ask God to help you see the spiritual lessons that He wants to teach you through these still, quiet times.

As you drive on a cross-country trip, you may see many warning signs: "Falling Rocks," "Do Not Enter," "Road Closed," "Keep Off," "Dead End" and so forth. God gives us warning signs in His Word. Observe the warning signs as you travel the pathway to success.

➼ According to the following Scriptures, what are the warnings that will help you on the pathway to success?

- Proverbs 4:14-19

- Proverbs 6:16-19

- Proverbs 22:24-25

- 1 Corinthians 10:12

Warning signs may be ignored until we discover the harsh reality of not obeying. The consequences may be lifelong. We too often ignore warning signs concerning our health. Daily the media tell us the benefits of a diet based on grains, fresh fruits, vegetables and lean meat. We have constant warnings about the results of a life without regular exercise. Yet many of us continue our unhealthy lifestyle until we have a serious physical problem. God's Word reminds us of the wisdom of listening to warnings.

➤ Read the following selections from Proverbs that remind us of the wisdom of instruction. Write any of these instructions that you feel speak to your life today.

- Proverbs 4:13

- Proverbs 13:13

- Proverbs 19:20

 Father God, as I read and study Your Word, help me to heed the warning signs so that I might be on guard and prepared to deal with life's dangers.

DAY 4: *Police Officers*

Cindy saw the flashing lights of a police car in her rearview mirror. Immediately, she pulled over and prepared to stop. Her heart beat a little faster. Adrenaline rushed through her bloodstream. Fortunately, the officer raced past her. Cindy wondered why she had reacted defensively. Don't overlook the important role of the police officers that God sends to offer instruction and correction along life's highways.

➤ According to Hebrews 13:17, what does God expect from us regarding our leaders?

➤ According to Romans 13:1, why must we obey the authorities?

⇒ According to 1 Peter 2:13-17, how does obeying authority affect our witness to the world?

⇒ According to Colossians 1:16-17, who created all powers, rulers and authorities?

⇒ In Titus 3:1-2, what did Paul tell Titus to remind the people of in regard to rulers and authorities?

The law-enforcement officers and other authority figures God places in our lives are not to be feared; rather, they are to be respected and appreciated, for they serve as protectors, counselors, defenders and directors in our lives. God uses other people to instruct and correct us. Follow the guidance of those God sends into your life, including your First Place leader.

⇒ Are you a good follower? Explain.

 Loving Father God, show me how to reap the benefits of following those You have put in authority over me. Thank You for my First Place leader, my pastor and others whom I depend upon for leadership.

DAY 5: Yield Signs

Yielding requires giving the right-of-way to someone else. Spiritually, we are to yield to God's authority in our lives. Through yielding, we recognize who is in charge and give Him control of our lives. Then we can safely proceed in the right direction.

In the following Scriptures, to what and to whom are we to yield?

- Matthew 7:21-23

- Matthew 10:37-39

- Matthew 16:24-26

Everything about us, everything we own, everyone we love—all must be yielded to God. Perhaps this explains why so many people do not stay on the pathway to success. Our human nature does not easily yield itself to the way of another, but yielding to God is the only way to successfully stay on track.

What is something or someone you have not yielded to God? Why?

Here are some examples of yielding to God's leadership through the First Place commitments: Take a walk instead of watching television; choose a fruit instead of a cookie; get up and do your Bible study instead of pushing the snooze alarm; memorize Scripture instead of listening to the car radio.

What yield sign has the Holy Spirit brought to your mind recently?

 Lord, I want to stay on track to success, and so I commit myself to live Your way. I know the only way to accomplish this is by being completely yielded to You. So, Father, I ask for renewed zeal for Your will in my life today, and that You would grace me to be willing to give everything to You.

DAY 6: *Reflections*

Staying on track to success has been the theme for this week's study. We have learned many things that can help us stay on track. The conclusion of Day 5 urged us to stay on track by committing ourselves to live God's way and showed us that the only way to live God's way is through being yielded completely to God. Completely yielded! How do we do this? The way to be completely yielded to God's way is to follow the example of Christ. So much of what Jesus did when He walked on this earth can be summarized by the word "yielded." Jesus was able to stay on track with the Father's plan because He daily chose to yield His will to that of the Father's. The same can be true of our lives, if we will choose to follow Christ and yield our will minute by minute, day by day, to the will of the Father.

John 4:31-34 reveals the yielded heart of Jesus and His commitment to staying on track and finishing the course His Father had planned for His life. Jesus spent time in prayer each day. He knew the Scriptures. He knew God's heart and He understood God's will—God's purpose and plan for His life. His power to live an earthly life that was yielded to the Father came from prayer, Scripture memory, Scripture reading and Bible study—all of which can empower each of us to yield our lives and will to the Father and help us to understand His purpose and plan. What food truly nourishes you today? Is it to do His will and to finish His work in your life?

 Father God, let me heed the words of Jesus: "I am the way and the truth and the life. No one comes to the Father except through me" (John 14:6). Lord, I realize that Jesus lived out a perfect example for me to follow, that He is the way, that He is the truth. I want to follow His example and live my life yielded to You. Thank You for sending Jesus to show me the way.

Heavenly Father, help me to daily heed the words of Joshua, who told the people to "throw away" the foreign gods, the idols that were among them, and to yield their hearts to the Lord, the God of Israel. And Lord, let my response be the same as when the people said to Joshua, "We will serve the LORD our God and obey him" (Joshua 24:24). Lord, I choose to serve You and to yield my heart and will to You. Let this be the food that I long to eat; let it satisfy my soul.

Lord, help me to keep my eyes straight ahead, to fix my gaze directly before me. Make level paths for my feet and strengthen me to take only the ways that are firm. Help me to not swerve to the right or the left; keep my feet from evil (see Proverbs 4:25-27).[1]

Lord, when You spoke to the children of Israel through Your prophet Jeremiah, You also had a message for Christians throughout all time. Thank You for Your written Word, which says that we will be Your people and You will be our God. Thank You for the promise that You will give us singleness of heart and action so that we will always fear and respect You. You said that this is for our own good and the good of our children after us. You have told us that You will make an everlasting covenant with Your people. You will never stop doing good to us, and You will inspire us to fear You, to worship and adore You, so we will never turn away from You (see Jeremiah 32:38-40).

DAY 7: *Reflections*

As we walk the paths of life and seek to stay on track to success, each of us will at one time or another encounter crossroads—times when we face a decision about which direction we should take or times when the circumstances of life change the course of our life. Relying on God when we encounter crossroads will enable us to steer our course safely on to our ultimate destination, to the realization of our goals and dreams, and to the completion of the plans and purposes God has for our lives.

As you conclude this week's study, review the memory verse for the week and then seek God's power and wisdom to guide you through the crossroads in your life.

 Lord Jehovah, in days of old You said to the people, "Stand at the crossroads and look; ask for the ancient paths, ask where the good way is, and walk in it, and you will find rest for your souls." But the people responded by saying, "We will not walk in it" (see Jeremiah 6:16). Father, when Jeremiah brought Your message to the people of Israel, they did not respond as they should have. Today, I have heard Your words in my heart and I want to have a different response. Help me to stop and look when I face crossroads in my life. Give me a heart determined to ask for the ancient paths, the paths that are well trodden by faithful men and women of God. I want to be one who will ask, "Where is the good way?" When You show me the way I am to go, O Lord, let my response always be, "Yes, I will walk in it."

"Show me your ways, O LORD, teach me your paths; guide me in your truth and teach me, for you are God my Savior, and my hope is in you all day long" (Psalm 25:4-5).[2] You are the only hope I have, Lord. Your path is the one that will keep me on track. Help me to follow You.

Lord, guard my course and protect my way as I pursue a righteous, victorious life in You (see Proverbs 2:8).[3] Be my strength when I am weak. Be my navigator and direct me each day. With Your almighty power to help me, Lord, I can keep going in the right direction. Help me to continue to follow the commitments, Lord, as I know You are using them to lead me to victory. When I fall down, help me get up again.

You, Lord, give strength to the weary and increase the power of the weak. You say that even those who are young grow tired and weary, and young men stumble and fall. But all those who hope in You, Lord, will renew their strength. We will soar on wings like eagles; we will run and not grow weary; we will walk and not be faint (see Isaiah 40:29-31). Father, when I am weary of the journey, I will wait on You. I will remember these verses. I will not take the wrong path and give up. I will stay on track and wait for You to renew my strength. Let me soar like an eagle, Lord!

Notes

1. Beth Moore, *Praying God's Word* (Nashville, TN: Broadman and Holman, 2000), p. 295.
2. Ibid., p. 75.
3. Ibid., p. 295.

Group Prayer Requests Today's Date:_____

Name	Request	Results

MANAGING SUCCESS

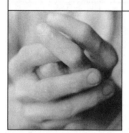

MEMORY VERSE
Guard the good deposit that was entrusted
to you—guard it with the help of the
Holy Spirit who lives in us.
2 Timothy 1:14

When Cindy reached her first weight goal, she was ecstatic! Overcoming the urge to treat herself to a chocolate milk shake, Cindy celebrated by going to a movie. The next goal did not seem so ominous. However, instead of more success, Cindy found herself plateauing. The weight loss stopped. Cindy needed to learn to manage her initial success, so that one goal led to accomplishing another. In this week's study we will concentrate on building on the success you have achieved thus far in First Place.

DAY 1: *Guard Against Pride—Cultivate Humility*

When you began to experience some measure of success in your lifestyle choices, who did you thank? Guard against a prideful, arrogant spirit. Pride is the sin of self-sufficiency. Pride leads us to think *I am adequate within myself.* It fails to acknowledge the source of our blessings—God Himself— and uses these blessings in a self-centered way.

➣ According to Deuteronomy 8:10-14, why can success be dangerous?

➣ After reading Psalm 10:4, check the answer that best completes the following statement: The problem with pride is that

      ☐ It makes us feel good about ourselves and our accomplishments.
      ☐ It gives the credit to self and not to God.

Success should encourage and motivate us to continue to improve ourselves. Feeling positive about yourself is not the sin of pride. Pride robs God of the credit for every good gift from above (see James 1:17).

➣ According to Proverbs 16:18-19, what does pride lead to?

Prayerfully ask God to help guard your heart from an arrogant, haughty pride. In your prayer journal, list the blessings in your life for which you want to give God the credit. Praise Him for each one!

A spirit of humility will guard our hearts from becoming filled with pride and arrogance. Cindy struggled with pride because of the attention she received from losing weight. When she began to realize that ungodly pride resided in her heart, Cindy knew she needed to develop a spirit of humility. She began to pray daily for God's help.

➣ Picture yourself kneeling before the Father. Draw or describe this picture of humility.

➣ Match the following verses with God's actions toward those who are humble:

_____ Psalm 18:27	a.	He exalts.
_____ Psalm 25:9	b.	He sustains.
_____ Psalm 147:6	c.	He saves.
_____ Matthew 23:12	d.	He gives grace.
_____ 1 Peter 5:5-6	e.	He guides.

Luke 18:9-14 records a parable that Jesus told to teach the difference between self-righteousness and humility.

➤ How would you characterize persons with a

Self-righteous attitude?

Humble attitude?

➤ After reading Philippians 2:5-8, describe the humility of Jesus.

Christ is our perfect example of humility. He laid aside His divinity and His royalty to put on the form of a man. In humility, He willingly suffered and gave His life on the cross. His humility allows us the opportunity of eternal life. In humility, we accept His gift of salvation.

➤ How will a spirit of humility help you maintain success in First Place?

➤ How will a lack of humility affect your success in First Place?

Begin reviewing the memory verse for this week and as you do, remember to thank God for helping you to memorize His Word throughout this study. Continue to review memory verses from previous weeks.

 Lord God, search my heart and reveal to me what You see. I humble myself before You.

DAY 2: *Avoid Envy and Jealousy*

Cindy often found herself resenting the success of others. The men in her group lost weight much faster than the women. And they were allowed more calories!

The success of others can sometimes be difficult on our ego. Like Cindy, are you envious of someone in your group? Is your jealousy affecting your relationships with others? Perhaps your success has been a source of envy for someone else. God's Word can help us learn to cope with the success of others as well as our own success.

➤ According to Galatians 5:24-26, what have those who belong to Christ Jesus put to death?

➤ What are they to live by?

➤ What are they instructed not to do?

➤ According to James 3:14-16, envy is earthly, unspiritual and comes from _____, not from heaven.

➤ What is found where envy and selfish ambition exist?

➤ Read Romans 1:29; Galatians 5:19-21; 1 Peter 2:1. Envy is listed in the same company with what other sins?

➤ Read 1 Corinthians 13:1-13 (read in the *New Living Translation*, if available). Write verse 4.

To avoid envy and jealousy, Cindy needed to learn about agape love—God's kind of love as described in 1 Corinthians 13. Cindy began to pray for God to change her heart and to teach her to understand and practice agape love.

 Lord, please heal me of any envy or jealousy I may feel. I ask that You would instill in me a love like Yours so that I am able to manage the success of others and to love others with a pure heart.

DAY 3: *Plug In to Your Power Source*

To manage her success in a godly manner, Cindy needed to give God the credit. She needed to remember that the things she had accomplished did not result from her own strength. It was God who had given her the power and strength to lose weight and to develop a more balanced life spiritually, mentally, emotionally and physically.

How easy it is for us to forget the source of our power to succeed! Our sinful nature deceives us, tricking us into believing we succeed on our own strength. The Bible is quick to remind us of the grace that is liberally poured out on us from God. Do you remember where your source of power comes from?

➤ After reading John 15:1-5, draw lines to complete the following analogies:

God is   the branch.

Jesus is   the gardener/pruner.

The believer is   the vine.

➤ What is the result when believers remain in (connect with) Jesus?

☐ They grow and produce fruit.

☐ They are pruned.

☐ They are cast in the fire.

➤ What is an area in your life God is seeking to prune (or cleanse)?

➤ According to Ephesians 3:20, what is God's power able to do in you?

As you continue on the pathway to success, remember that God is your source of power. If you try to rely on your own strength, you will eventually run out of the will and motivation to keep going. If you are leaning on someone else besides God for strength, he or she will not always be there. God's abundant grace is much more powerful. Thank Him today for being your source of power.

 Father God, thank You that You are a loving gardener who prunes to help me produce more abundantly. Help me, Lord, to rely on You for the power and grace I need to change or remove those things that drag me from Your path to success.

DAY 4: *Share the Good News*

As you experience God's power in your life and success in First Place, you will want to share your testimony with others. People need encouragement in the area of weight management and nutrition. Many need hope. Others need to know how to develop a daily walk with Christ. Are you prepared to share your testimony with others?

➤ Read Luke 8:26-39 and then briefly describe the condition of the man Jesus encountered.

> What did Jesus do for the man?

> What did Jesus tell the man to do?

> How did the man respond to Jesus' instructions?

Briefly scan John 4:4-30, the story of the woman at the well. What did the woman declare about Jesus (v. 29)?

> Name someone with whom you want to share the good news that "this is the Christ."

God can use your personal testimony to help bring others to Himself and give hope to the hopeless. Write your First Place testimony in your prayer journal or on a separate piece of paper. Answering the following questions will help you as you write:

- What was your condition when you started First Place? (May include physical, emotional, mental and spiritual condition.)

- What has Jesus done for you? How has your life been changed?

- How has your life been affected by keeping the nine First Place commitments?

- What is your condition at the present time? What have you learned?

Thank God that you have good news to share! Ask for boldness to share your testimony with someone else this week. Take time to consider the encouragement commitment and contact someone new this week. Is there a fellow class member who needs a word of encouragement or praise? Send a note or call someone today. Ask what God has done in his or her life during this session.

Anyone with good manners has learned the value of the simple expression "thank you." As you learn to manage success, remember to praise God for all He has done for you. Thank Him now. Allow Him to receive the glory and honor due His name for the mighty wonders He is performing in your life.

To get the story, a good reporter learns to ask why, what, when and how. Answer these questions as you read the following Scriptures:

➣ Psalm 100:4-5—Why are we to praise God?

➣ Hebrews 13:15—When are we to praise God?

➣ 1 Peter 1:3-4—What are we to praise God for?

➣ Read Psalm 150; Jude 24-25 and Revelation 4:11. How are we to praise God?

➣ Evaluate the degree to which praise is a part of your life by placing an X on the following continuum:

1	2	3	4	5
Not characteristic			Highly characteristic	

In managing success, remember to praise God and give Him all the credit. We also can thank our First Place leader(s) and fellow group members, as well as family and friends who have helped us. We can even pat ourselves on the back a little for staying with the program, but God is the One who has empowered and helped us succeed.

> Write a prayer of thanksgiving and praise to God. Give Him all the glory for the things He has done during this session of First Place. Offer Him a heart filled with praise and glory for all He has done. Thank Him in advance for the things He will do in the future, as You continue to give Him first place in your life.

DAY 5: *Move On to New Goals*

Enjoying our success, reveling in victories and achievements, is wonderfully satisfying. It is an experience well earned and well deserved, a time to cherish. However, if we linger in this time of celebration too long, we can become stagnant and complacent—or even regress. When we complete a goal or see our dreams come to fruition, we need new direction. Seeking God's heart for new dreams will help us maintain the success we have enjoyed and propel us forward to new opportunities.

> After reading again the *King James Version* of the memory verse from week one, Proverbs 29:18, recall why we need a vision, goal or dream.

The apostle Paul must have understood the need to move on to new goals.

➤ Read Philippians 3:13-14 and rewrite the verses in your own words.

➤ Are you willing to move forward by setting new goals?

☐ Yes   ☐ No

What are the desires of your heart? In your prayer journal, write any dreams or goals God places in your heart. Courageously step out in faith that He will help you succeed in anything He calls you to do. You may want to review week two, "Plan for Success."

➤ List one new goal. Or you may want to list a goal still in progress. Remember that a long-range goal must include short-range goals that will move you closer to accomplishing it.

Dear Lord, I commit my dreams and goals to You. Grace me to walk in faithful and steadfast obedience. I trust in Your almighty power and strength to accomplish Your plans in me.

DAY 6: *Reflections*

Week nine has brought us to a place of contemplation and self-evaluation. We have been presented with several ideas that can help us to manage success. However small or great the measure of success may be, it is to be managed in a godly manner. We are challenged to consider the questions: *How do I handle success?* and *How do I handle the success of others?*

Review the ways to manage success that we have studied this week.

- 🍎 Guard against pride.
- 🍎 Cultivate humility.
- 🍎 Avoid envy and jealousy.
- 🍎 Plug in to your power source.
- 🍎 Share the good news.
- 🍎 Praise and glorify God.
- 🍎 Move on to new goals.

Did you notice anything unique about the list? Each one of these begins with a verb—an action word. Managing success requires action on our part; it doesn't just happen on its own. We must prepare our minds and hearts to act so as to give a godly response to success; taking action on the things we learned this week will help us to do that.

Father, help me to clothe myself with humility toward others, because You oppose the proud but give grace to the humble (see 1 Peter 5:5). I will never live a day that I am not in need of Your grace, so please help me maintain an attitude that welcomes it.[1]

Father, according to Your Word, in their pride the wicked do not seek You; in all their thoughts there is no room for You (see Psalm 10:4). Please help me to always make room in my thoughts for You, God. Don't allow me to continue on in pride that stops me from seeking You.[2]

Father, Your Word tells me that You rebuke the arrogant, those who are cursed and who stray from Your commands (see Psalm 119:21). Keep my heart humble, Lord. Let me always remember that You are the one who has given me success. Let me never try to take credit that belongs to You. Without You, Lord, I could not have any freedom and victory in my life.

Mighty God, deliverer of my soul, You say that before his downfall a man's heart is proud, but humility comes before honor (see Proverbs 18:12). By Your great power and Your incredible goodness toward me, I have walked this pathway to success and made progress along the way. I praise You for all that You have done. Please forbid any hint of ungodly pride to swell up in my heart and cause my downfall. Fill me with genuine humility. Let me never forget my source of power—You, Lord; keep me plugged in to You.

Glorious Lord, with a grateful heart I pray in agreement with the words of the psalmist, who said, "I will praise you, O LORD, with all my heart; I will tell of all your wonders. I will be glad and rejoice in you; I will sing praise to your name, O Most High" (Psalm 9:1-2). Father, be with me when I share the good news of what You have done in my life during this session, for I want to give You all the praise and glory.

DAY 7: Reflections

Our study this week on managing success is likely challenging to each one of us in one way or another. While one may struggle with pride, another may struggle with envy or jealousy, and someone else may fear sharing his or her testimony. Others may fear moving on to a new goal. Any one of us could forget to thank the Lord for what He has done in our lives. We could even begin to drift away from the source of our power, the Lord. God knows our hearts. If we truly want to manage success in a godly manner, His Spirit and His Word will provide the help we need. How does success affect you? What is your response to success?

Review your memory verse and, as you pray today, thank God for the good deposit He has given you to guard; thank Him for the Holy Spirit who helps you to guard it. Then, allow the following outline to be the foundation of your time of prayer today (choose one or more, or all, of the points of the outline):

Ask God to search your heart.

"Search me, O God, and know my heart; test me and know my anxious thoughts. See if there is any offensive way in me, and lead me in the way everlasting" (Psalm 139:23-24). Father, if I fail to see any negative, ungodly response to success in myself, I ask You to reveal it to me and to teach me to manage success rightly. Lord, anytime I face challenges or strongholds in my life, search my heart and lead me to Your pathways.

Abide with God and fellow believers.

"Let us draw near to God with a sincere heart in full assurance of faith, having our hearts sprinkled to cleanse us from a guilty conscience and having our bodies washed with pure water. Let us hold unswervingly to the hope we profess, for he who promised is faithful. And let us consider how we may spur one another on toward love and good deeds. Let us not give up meeting together, as some are in the habit of doing, but let us encourage one another—and all the more as you see the Day approaching" (Hebrews 10:22-25). Father, give me a heart that longs to be in Your presence. Give me a passion for You, Lord. Help our group to draw close to each other and encourage one another to continue on the pathway to success.

Accept God's grace and His commands.

"For it is by grace you have been saved, through faith—and this not from yourselves, it is the gift of God—not by works, so that no one can boast. For we are God's workmanship, created in Christ Jesus to do good works, which God prepared in advance for us to do" (Ephesians 2:8-10). "I have sought your face with all my heart; be gracious to me according to your promise. I have considered my ways and have turned my steps to your statutes. I will hasten and not delay to obey your commands" (Psalm 119:58-60). Sovereign and merciful Lord, I confess to You that I have fallen short in managing success. I accept Your promised gift of grace, by faith, and ask You to help me follow Your commands. Remove any hint of boastfulness and pride from my heart, Lord.

Aspire to reflect God's character.

"Therefore, prepare your minds for action; be self-controlled; set your hope fully on the grace to be given you when Jesus Christ is revealed. As obedient children, do not conform to the evil desires you had when you lived in ignorance. But just as he who called you is holy, so be holy in all you do; for it is written: 'Be holy, because I am holy'" (1 Peter 1:13-16). Almighty God, You have been at work in my heart this week helping me to see my responses to success, and even my responses to a lack of success in a few areas. You have helped me to evaluate my heart and mind—You have corrected my footsteps and brought me back on course. Thank You for teaching me how to manage success. I pray that You will help me to take action and follow through on what I have learned. Teach me to reflect Your character more each day. I still have a long way to go, but I know that You will be with me each step.

Always give God the credit.

 "Give thanks to the LORD, call on his name; make known among the nations what he has done. Sing to him, sing praise to him; tell of all his wonderful acts. Glory in his holy name; let the hearts of those who seek the LORD rejoice. Look to the LORD and his strength; seek his face always. Remember the wonders he has done, his miracles, and the judgments he pronounced, O descendants of Abraham his servant, O sons of Jacob, his chosen ones" (Psalm 105:1-6). Father, with all my heart I want to give praise and glory to Your name and to thank You for helping me on this journey. Let me never take credit that belongs to You. Thank You for the victories You have given me along the way. Let me not forget what You have done.

Notes
1. Beth Moore, *Praying God's Word* (Nashville, TN: Broadman and Holman, 2000), p. 67.
2. Ibid., p. 61.

GROUP PRAYER REQUESTS   TODAY'S DATE:_____

NAME	REQUEST	RESULTS

CALLED
TO SUCCESS!

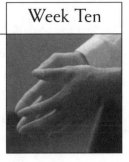

MEMORY VERSE

*You are a chosen people, a royal priesthood, a holy
nation, a people belonging to God, that you may
declare the praises of him who called you out of
darkness into his wonderful light.*

1 Peter 2:9

With God's help, Cindy did succeed in achieving her long-term goal of
losing 100 pounds. Along the way, she made many wise lifestyle choices
and grew significantly as a Christian. Today Cindy is a First Place leader,
helping others follow the pathway to success. As a child of the King, as a
royal champion empowered by Christ, you too can succeed at your goals.
You are called to success!

DAY 1: *Choose Blessings*

When Cindy began First Place, she made a wise choice. Instead of eating
a big meal at the end of the day, she ate smaller portions throughout the
day. She chose to exercise three to five days each week by walking the
track in the family life center of her church. Cindy chose to take time to
read God's Word, to pray and to do her Bible study. Lifestyle changes are
made choice by choice, day by day! We have freedom of choice. When
we choose life in Christ, we can experience God's blessings for ourselves
and others.

> According to Deuteronomy 30:19-20, what choices did God set
> before the Israelites?

⋙ What blessings were promised if they made wise choices?

Many of life's circumstances cannot be altered, but we can be royal champions in spite of a difficult situation. When we choose wisely, we can claim God's blessings.

⋙ How does the First Place program represent a choice that brings life instead of death?

The pathway to success leads to a glorious destination for those who are called and for those who then choose blessings by choosing to walk with God. Consider this thought: *Although we have been called to success, we must do our part.* God doesn't just cause us to succeed without our doing our part. To travel the path of life and experience God's greatest blessings, we must

🍎 Choose to answer His voice when He calls.

🍎 Choose to accept His invitation to walk with Him.

🍎 Choose to act on what He teaches us in His Word and through others.

🍎 Choose to adhere to His path.

🍎 Choose to attain the prize by diligently pressing on to the prize to which He is calling us heavenward (see Philippians 3:14).

⋙ Are you choosing to do your part?

☐ Yes　　☐ No

⋙ Do you believe that God will do His part?

☐ Yes　　☐ No

Doing our part is a daily process. Cindy learned that God blessed her life in many different ways as she daily chose to do her part. When she stumbled and fell, she sought God's forgiveness for her poor choices, and then by His grace she started again. She discovered that God is always faithful to do His part and that the Holy Spirit's power would help her to do hers.

Ask forgiveness for ways you have chosen death (unhealthy lifestyle choices) over life. Begin anew to choose God's ways and receive His blessings. Choose life by faithfully committing God's Word to memory. Daily, choose to do your part; daily, trust God to do His. Begin learning the memory verse for this week by writing the verse in your prayer journal. Frequently review previous memory verses by listening to all of the verses on the Scripture Memory Music CD and by using *Walking in the Word*.

 Heavenly Father, forgive me for ways I have chosen death over life by making unhealthy lifestyle choices. I desire to begin anew to choose Your ways and receive Your blessings. God, I choose life by faithfully committing Your Word to memory, and I daily choose to do my part and trust You to do Yours.

DAY 2: *Decide to Change*

When God chose us as His holy nation, He called us out of darkness. As surely as a caterpillar changes into a beautiful butterfly, you too can be a new creation in Christ. Make the necessary changes to achieve your goals and become a royal champion.

In Ephesians 4:21-24, Paul wrote that we are to be made new by the attitudes of our mind.

➤ What corrupts the old self that would be changed by the new attitudes of our mind?

➤ The new self is created to be like God in true _____ and_____.

➤ List some examples of the old self that you have put off.

➤ List some new attitudes you have put on.

Righteousness refers to our right standing with God, which results in right living. Holiness means being set apart from the world's ways for service to God.

Read Colossians 3:12-17. The following is a list of the characteristics that God's chosen people should clothe themselves in.

➤ Have you changed into these garments? Check all that you currently wear as a chosen child, a royal champion of the King, called to the pathway of success.

☐ Compassion ☐ Gentleness

☐ Kindness ☐ Patience

☐ Humility ☐ Love

➤ Which one of these virtues binds all the others together in perfect unity?

➤ According to verse 15, what is to rule our hearts?

➤ Write verse 16 in your own words.

➤ What does Paul say in verse 17 that would cause you to decide to make changes in the things you do?

➤ Check the response that best describes you now.

☐ I am wearing the old self.

☐ I am changing to the new self.

☐ I have put on the new self.

We can choose to walk in victory as children of the risen King of kings who will give us the power to change. Have you put on your purple robe of royalty? Or are you still wearing your old rags?

Prayerfully consider aspects of your old self that need to change in order for you to succeed. List one change that you will work on today, and write a prayer asking God to empower you to make that change.

DAY 3: *Stand Firm and Defeat the Darkness*

Adverse circumstances, trials and temptations can cause us to lose our firm footing, which can affect our potential for success and perhaps make us doubt that we have been called to success. Relying on God's faithfulness, we can stand on the firm foundation, Jesus Christ our cornerstone.

➤ According to Matthew 7:24-27, when adverse circumstances came, what happened to the foolish man?

➤ What happened to the wise man?

❧ According to this parable, who is wise?

Avoid placing confidence in your own abilities and efforts. Paul said, "If you think you are standing firm, be careful that you don't fall" (1 Corinthians 10:12).

In Philippians 3:18—4:1, Paul told us how to stand firm in the Lord.

❧ Draw a connecting line to correctly describe the characteristics of those who do not stand firm.

Their glory	is in their shame.
They are enemies	is destruction.
Their destiny	of the Cross.
Their god	is their stomach.

❧ Those who stand firm eagerly await _____.

This passage helped Cindy learn to stand firm by reminding her to keep her focus on Jesus and her mind on things above rather than on earthly things. Allow these verses, and others that God shows you, to help you.

❧ According to 2 Thessalonians 2:15, what is another way to stand firm?

When adverse circumstances, trials or temptations come into your life and cause you to lose your balance or to even stumble and fall, you can find help to regain your footing. You can learn how to stand firm by keeping your eyes on Jesus and making Him your sure foundation. Remember, you are a royal champion, a child of the almighty King of kings who has already won the victory on your behalf. Pause and thank the Lord for being your sure foundation and for His teachings that help you stand firm!

This week's memory verse declares that God called us out of darkness into His wonderful light. We are wise to be afraid of the dark when it represents the power of evil around us. Shine a small flashlight into a dark room. Notice how even the tiniest beam of light dispels a room full of darkness.

Consider John 1:6-8—John the Baptist came to witness to the light, Jesus Christ, who would give light to every person in the world. In John 8:12, Jesus affirmed John the Baptist's prophecy by declaring, "I am." Jesus' light dispels the darkness of evil; His light is the guiding light on our path.

➤ After reading 1 John 1:5-7, contrast people who walk in darkness with those who live in the light.

Darkness   Light

As a review from week four, read Ephesians 6:10-18. Wearing the whole armor of God will help us to defeat the darkness and allow us to be victorious royal champions.

Do you walk in the light? Today, as you have your quiet time, remember we can defeat the enemy if we live as children of the light. Spend a few minutes reviewing the memory verse, and faithfully read God's Word each day. Let the light of Christ shine through you!

 Thank You, Almighty God, for calling me out of the darkness and into Your glorious light. Help me to live as a child of the light, a child of the King.

DAY 4: *Never Give Up*

At times we may feel as though we cannot go on. We can become so weary of all that life demands of us. On more than one occasion, Cindy grew weary. At times she felt hopeless and as though the pathway to success must be meant for others in her group but not for her. We must never give in to fatigue that would lead us to give up on our goals.

≫ Write Galatians 6:9 in your own words.

≫ When will we reap this harvest—the fruit of our labors?

≫ What does this verse mean to you when considered in light of your First Place goals?

≫ What will reaping a harvest mean when applied to your First Place goals?

≫ What happens to you when your soul grows weary, as the psalmist described in Psalm 119:28?

Weary times are inevitable. We must be on guard at such times, allowing God to strengthen us according to His Word.

≫ According to 2 Timothy 1:12, what did Paul say encouraged him when times were hard?

He knew_____and he trusted_____

_____.

God used two things to encourage Cindy to persevere. He used the encouragement of others through their prayers, notes and calls. And He encouraged Cindy by His Spirit as she prayed, as she read His promises in the Scriptures, as she learned about the many accounts of men and women throughout the Bible who didn't give up, and as she listened to Christian hymns and praise music. What encourages you when you grow weary?

➤ What, if anything, are you weary of, or ready to give up on?

➤ Read Isaiah 40:28-31 and record God's promise to those who are weary.

➤ Recall a time in the past when you persevered, even though you wanted to give up.

Consider anyone in your group who may be weary or feels like giving up; pray for that person. If someone in the group has missed the last few meetings, decide to contact him or her today and encourage him or her to attend the meeting this week. Ask God to use you to encourage someone else. Following through with the encouragement commitment can make a difference! Send a note or call someone today who needs to stay on the path.

If you feel like giving up, ask the Lord to renew your spirit and your commitment. Ask Him to empower you to persevere on the path of success, the path of a victorious royal champion.

 Today, Heavenly Father, I commit to remain on the path to which You have called me—the pathway of success, my path as a chosen child of You, my King. In the glory of Your presence I will find strength to carry on.

DAY 5: *Cross the Finish Line and Claim Your Successes*

The finish line is the culmination of a race. How sad it is when an athlete is injured and unable to complete a race. There are many types of finish lines in the course of life—graduating from high school, finishing college or a trade school, completing a project at work and so forth. Whether achieving a goal in First Place, completing a special project or making it through an especially difficult day, don't let the enemy rob you of the satisfaction and joy of crossing the finish line.

➤ According to Paul's testimony in 2 Timothy 4:7-8, what was his reward for finishing the race?

➤ Referring to Hebrews 12:1-2, who are the ones witnessing your race?

➤ What things are hindering you from completing the race?

➤ Check all statements that describe how you are running your race.

☐ With hesitation in your steps
☐ With perseverance
☐ With confusion and no sense of direction
☐ With patience and fortitude
☐ With eyes on another runner
☐ With purpose in every step
☐ With hope and confidence in God
☐ With sin-entagled feet
☐ With your eyes on the goal
☐ With commitment and effort
☐ With awareness of the cloud of witnesses
☐ With determination to cross the finish line

➤ Are you running *your* race or trying to run the one marked out for someone else?

At the encouragement of a friend, Cindy entered a 10-K run. She was not a highly trained, fast-paced long-distance runner. She only jogged two to three miles per day at a medium pace, four to five days each week. The 10-K race would be a challenge. She decided that her primary goal would be to complete the course, no matter how long it took. She trained for many weeks before the race. She would compete against herself—no one else. Her family and friends would be waiting at the finish line. Before the race started, Cindy prayed and dedicated the race to the Lord, remembering the days before First Place when she was so severely overweight and out of shape that she couldn't jog at all. Cindy took the course at her own pace. Many runners passed her by and finished long before she did. But when she crossed the finish line with a sweaty brow, weary legs and tears of jubilation, the sound of cheers from those on the sideline rang in her ears. And, somehow, in her heart she felt that she could also hear the cheers and applause of her heavenly Father.

Someone is always watching and witnessing our achievements or failures, so don't give up. Your life can be a living testimony of the power of God; you can be an encouragement and inspire someone else as they run their race. Keep your eyes fixed on Jesus and the finish line ahead.

In your prayer journal, record your prayer of commitment to finishing the race, to succeed, to be a victorious royal champion.

➤ According to Philippians 1:6, who began the work in you?

➤ Who will finish the work in you?

➤ Are you confident that He will do it?

      ☐ Yes   ☐ No

Thomas Edison performed more than 2,000 experiments before he perfected a working lightbulb. He was asked how he felt about having failed so many times. Mr. Edison replied, "I never failed once. I invented the lightbulb. It just happened to be a 2,000-step process." Your success may be a 2,000-step process. Success is the *progressive* realization of your goals. Claim what God has already done in your life as you walk the pathway still ahead.

➤ Consider 1 Corinthians 9:24-25—are you running to win the prize (your goals)?

☐ Yes   ☐ No

➤ Read Psalm 20:4-5; what are the desires of your heart?

➤ Do you trust Him to make all your plans succeed?

☐ Yes   ☐ No

➤ Consider Deuteronomy 20:4—are you allowing the Lord to go with you in your daily battles?

☐ Yes   ☐ No

Have you seen victories in your daily life? Deuteronomy 20:4 tells us that the Lord God goes with us to fight against our enemies to give us victory.

➤ Recall the four areas of emphasis in First Place: spiritual, emotional, mental and physical. What progress have you seen in each of these areas?

➤ Of the following, check the evidences of growth that are true of you:

☐ Depending more on God and less on self
☐ Handling disruptions and disappointments without giving up
☐ Looking for ways to encourage and befriend others
☐ Exercising regularly
☐ Coming nearer to my ideal weight
☐ Memorizing Scripture
☐ Having regular quiet time
☐ Other(s)_____

➤ Record some of the successes (no matter how small) that God has given you as a victorious royal champion during this session of First Place.

Cindy had just completed a session as leader of a First Place group. A young man named Chuck in her group stayed to talk with her. He had not reached several of his goals for the session and was discouraged. "You don't know what it's like to try and try, yet see so little progress."

Cindy smiled. She thought about her days as a single parent, the nights in school after a long day's work, the self-esteem issues she had worked through. "I don't know when or how God will answer your prayers," Cindy told him. "Keeping Him first place in your life is more important than any other commitment. I know God is faithful."

As Chuck left the room, Cindy dropped to her knees, praising God for bringing her out of darkness into His wonderful light (see 1 Peter 2:9).

The pathway to success is not an accident. Daily you must choose to remain on the path. Always remember you are a royal champion, a son or daughter of the almighty Prince of Peace, who has already won the victory on your behalf. He has called you to success! You can succeed!

As you close this Bible study, meditate on this: "If God is for us, who can be against us? Who shall separate us from the love of Christ? Shall trouble or hardship or persecution or famine or nakedness or danger or sword? No, in all these things we are more than conquerors through him who loved us" (Romans 8:31,35,37).

Write a prayer of praise and thanksgiving to God for all He has done in your life this session, as well as all He will be doing in the future.

DAY 6: *Reflections*

As this session of this First Place study comes to a conclusion, take time to reflect on the pathway you have traveled. The chapter titles and memory verses are listed with a prayer for each. Consider the things God has done in your life through each week of this study. In your prayer journal, offer praises to Him for areas where you have experienced victory and growth, and seek His guidance in any areas where you still need His help. The things God has taught you in these 10 weeks are valuable lessons to take with you as you continue the journey on the pathway to success.

Week One: Dream of Success

"Where there is no vision, the people perish" (Proverbs 29:18, *KJV*). Almighty Lord, thank You for the visions and dreams that You have placed in my heart. You have given my life direction and purpose.

Week Two: Plan for Success

"May He give you the desire of your heart and make all your plans succeed" (Psalm 20:4). Gracious Father, You have walked with me these many weeks, and I can see that the desires of my heart and the plans we made together are beginning to become a reality in my life. Lord, to my surprise, some of the things I thought I wanted don't seem quite as important as they did 10 weeks ago. You have given me some new desires. I have discovered that knowing You more intimately and walking the path with You are the greatest desires of my heart.

Week Three: Surrender for Success

"Love the Lord your God with all your heart and with all your soul and with all your strength" (Deuteronomy 6:5). Lord, with all my heart, I want to love You completely. Help me to daily surrender my will and my life to You. Help me to surrender my affections and appetites. May my allegiance be to You above all else. Lord, please continue to teach me to surrender my attitudes and actions, and may they glorify You.

Father, help me to surrender all my anxieties and answers. Help me trust in You when I have worries and fears. Let me look to You when I need answers. Father, with each passing day may I have a heart that is more completely surrendered to You. May my heart and life always express true love and adoration for You.

Week Four: Dress for Success

"Put on the full armor of God so that you can take your stand against the devil's schemes" (Ephesians 6:11). Almighty God, You have told me to put on Your armor. Each day, I am trying to be faithful to do this, for I have realized that without Your armor, I am truly defenseless against Satan's schemes.

Thank You, Lord, for giving me the powerful weapon of Your Word! Help me to continue to memorize Scripture and to frequently review the verses I have learned during this session. With Your help, O Lord, I can stand against the enemy.

Week Five: Keys to Success

"His divine power has given us everything we need for life and godliness through our knowledge of him who called us by his own glory and goodness" (2 Peter 1:3). Father, thank You for Your power, the Holy Spirit who is mightily at work in me. Thank You for calling me to the path of life—to know You and to walk with You. Help me to grow in godliness with each step. You have taught me about many keys that, when combined with Your power, will help me to live a godly life. Thank You for each key, Lord.

Father, You have shown me that the pathway to success requires commitment and effort, honesty and integrity, wisdom and understanding, courage and strength, support and encouragement, patience and fortitude. You have shown me that obedience and blessings go hand in hand. May Your divine power and these keys continue to be at work in my heart long beyond the ending of this session.

Week Six: Thoughts That Build Success

"Search me, O God, and know my heart; test me and know my anxious thoughts. See if there is any offensive way in me, and lead me in the way everlasting" (Psalm 139:23-24). Father, You know my every thought, and You are well aware of how my thoughts so often sabotage me. Please continue to search my heart and rid me of any thoughts that hinder me from progressing on the path You have for me.

Lord, I want to learn to have a deeper confidence in You and to make wise choices each day. Give me a hopeful heart that believes You can do great and mighty things.

Father, help me to have healthy self-esteem by understanding how much You love me and that I am a new creation in Christ. Help me to be willing to be available to You. Let me have a mind-set that is persistent and optimistic. Lead me in the way You want me to go, Lord. Keep my thoughts on You.

Week Seven: Overcoming Leads to Success

"Everyone born of God overcomes the world. This is the victory that has overcome the world, even our faith. Who is it that overcomes the world? Only he who believes that Jesus is the Son of God" (1 John 5:4-5). O Lord, truly You have overcome this world. You have said that by faith in Your son, Christ Jesus, we overcome the world. Continue to build my faith and trust in You, Father. You are my banner of victory; lead me to success in overcoming habits, mistakes and sin, false expectations, willfulness, limitations, temptations and doubts.

Week Eight: Staying on Track to Success

"Whether you turn to the right or to the left, your ears will hear a voice behind you, saying, 'This is the way; walk in it'" (Isaiah 30:21). Father, help me to listen to You and to follow Your direction. Keep me on track, Lord, and help me not to stray from the course You have planned for my life.

Lord, let me keep my eyes and thoughts focused on You, the pathway to success, because everything in life surely gravitates toward that which my mind and thoughts are focused upon.

Week Nine: Managing Success

"Guard the good deposit that was entrusted to you—guard it with the help of the Holy Spirit who lives in us" (2 Timothy 1:14). O Lord, You have been so good to me and have given me so much during these past weeks. Let me carefully guard the treasured lessons and the victories You have given to me. Help me to guard against pride that fails to give You the glory. Help me to cultivate a spirit of humility and avoid envy and jealousy of others. Lord, let me not forget that You are the source of my power; let me abide in You always. Give me courage to share the good news of what You have done in my life, and may I always give the praise and glory to You. Continue Your work in me and give me new visions and new goals. Let Your Spirit fill me each day, giving me power to walk the path ahead.

Week Ten: Called to Success

"You are a chosen people, a royal priesthood, a holy nation, a people belonging to God, that you may declare the praises of him who called you out of darkness into his wonderful light" (1 Peter 2:9). Almighty God, thank You for calling me to be one of Your people, for calling me to be a royal champion, a child of the King of kings. Thank You for calling me out of the darkness and into Your light.

Father, I choose blessings and life in You. Give me Your power to change where I need to change and help me to stand firm on the Rock of my salvation, Jesus, who helps me to defeat the darkness. Let me be faithful to walk in the light, never giving up, but persevering to cross the finish line. Let me claim the victory that is mine in Christ Jesus. Let me proclaim what You have already done in my life as I continue to walk by faith, knowing that You have even greater successes ahead. Let me stay on the pathway to success till that day when I will see You face-to-face.

DAY 7: *Reflections*

This week's study brings us to a turning point on our pathway to success. It ends a 10-week Bible study, but the journey continues for all who have been called to follow the pathway to success. What is the pathway to success? It is far more than the accomplishment of our health and fitness goals or any number of other dreams and goals we desire to accomplish. Do you fear where the path may take you from here? The Bible tells of many who walked the path, of many who encountered turning points and continued on by trusting and obeying God. Consider just one example of the many recorded in God's Word—the words of the Lord to Joshua when he came to a turning point in his path:

> After the death of Moses the servant of the LORD, the LORD said to Joshua son of Nun, Moses' aide: "Moses my servant is dead. Now then, you and all these people, get ready to cross the Jordan River into the land I am about to give to them—to the Israelites. I will give you every place where you set your foot, as I promised Moses. As I was with Moses, so I will be with you; I will never leave you nor forsake you. Be strong and very courageous. Be careful to obey all the law my servant Moses gave you; do not turn from it to the right or to the left, that you may be successful wherever you go. Do not let this Book of the Law depart from your mouth; meditate on it day and night, so that you may be careful to do everything written in it. Then you will be prosperous and successful. Have I not commanded you? Be strong and courageous. Do not be terrified; do not be discouraged, for the LORD your God will be with you wherever you go" (Joshua 1:1-3,5,7-9).

The saints of old have walked the path before us. They followed the path God called them to walk. At times, they encountered trials and hardships, just as we will, but they walked in intimate fellowship with God through the good times and difficult times, till He called them to their heavenly home. We, too, must be strong, courageous and careful to obey God's Word. We don't need to be afraid of the path ahead, for He will be with us.

The little book titled *Success* quotes Roy Lessin's description of success:

Success is fulfilling the purpose for which something is made. A plane would be a failure if it couldn't fly; a boat would be a failure if it didn't float. Our highest purpose is to know God and be reflections of Him to others. When our feet are walking this path, we are on the high road to success.[1]

Knowing God and reflecting His glory is the true pathway to success. It is found in a daily walk, a commitment to a lifelong journey of walking in intimate fellowship with God through prayer, Bible study, Scripture reading, worship, praise, obedience, a vibrant growing faith and so much more. May it be the sincere desire of your heart to continue on the high road, the pathway to success.

Select from the following Scripture prayers as you begin your prayer time. Include a time of thanksgiving and praise for the things God has done in your life during these past 10 weeks. Ask the Father to give you a heart that is committed to continuing on the pathway to success. Ask Him to give you a hunger to know Him more and to allow you to be a radiant reflection of Him.

Lord Jehovah, when You saw that Moses had gone over to look at the burning bush, You, O God, called to him from within the bush, You called him by name, and Moses answered, "Here I am" (Exodus 3:4). Father, You are calling my name just as You did to Moses. With all my heart, Lord, this is my response: *Here I am.* Lord, I am choosing to answer You and accept Your invitation to know You and to walk with You. Help me to act on what I have learned and to be open to all that You will teach me in the future. Hold my feet to the path; I want to walk in Your light. Let me obey Your guidance and walk close to You, just as Moses did.

Gracious Lord, You give me Your shield of victory; You stoop down to make me great. You broaden the path beneath me, so that my ankles do not turn (see 2 Samuel 22:36-37). You have given me so many victories and blessings in my life through this study. Thank You, Father. Be near me as I continue on this journey.

You have made known to me the path of life; You will fill me with joy in Your presence, with eternal pleasures at Your right hand (see Psalm 16:11). Father, thank You for showing me the pathway of life and success. Thank You for allowing me to experience the joy of Your exquisite presence.

By faith Abraham, when called to go to a place he would later receive as his inheritance, obeyed and went, even though he did not know where he was going (see Hebrews 11:8). Father, help me to obey You, even though I don't always know what You have planned or where You are sending me.

Lord God, "Your word is a lamp to my feet and a light for my path" (Psalm 119:105). Teach me, O LORD, to follow Your decrees; then I will keep them to the end. "Give me under-standing, and I will keep your law and obey it with all my heart. Direct me in the path of your commands, for there I find delight" (Psalm 119:34-35). Father, "I have chosen the way of truth; I have set my heart on your laws. I hold fast to your statutes, O LORD; do not let me be put to shame. I run in the path of your commands, for you have set my heart free" (Psalm 119:30-32).

Lord, God, how I pray that You may count me worthy of Your calling and that by Your power You may fulfill every good purpose of mine and every act prompted by my faith (see 2 Thessalonians 1:11).[2]

"For this reason I kneel before the Father, from whom his whole family in heaven and on earth derives its name. I pray that out of his glorious riches he may strengthen [me] with power through his Spirit in [my] inner being, so that Christ may dwell in [my heart] through faith. And I pray that [I], being rooted and established in love, may have power, together with all the saints, to grasp how wide and long and high and deep is the love of Christ, and to know this love that surpass-es knowledge—that [I] may be filled to the measure of all the fullness of God. Now to him who is able to do immeasurably more than all [I] ask or imagine, according to his power that is at work within [me], to him be glory in the church and in Christ Jesus throughout all generations, for ever and ever! Amen" (Ephesians 3:14-21).

Notes

1. Roy Lessin, quoted in Scott Kennedy, *Success* (Bloomington, MN: Garborg's Heart and Home, Inc., 1997), n.p.

2. Beth Moore, *Praying God's Word* (Nashville, TN: Broadman and Holman, 2000), p. 51.

GROUP PRAYER REQUESTS   TODAY'S DATE:_____

NAME	REQUEST	RESULTS

ADDING FLAVOR
THE HEALTHY WAY

SODIUM/SALT

When it comes to health, sodium (salt) has drawn a considerable amount of attention because of its relationship to high blood pressure. High blood pressure is a leading risk factor for heart attack, stroke and kidney disease. Scientists have discovered that some people's blood pressure is very sensitive to excess sodium in the diet. Because high blood pressure is such a serious health problem, the current U.S. Dietary Guidelines call for Americans to choose a diet moderate in salt and sodium.

Sodium Requirements

Currently, there is no Recommended Dietary Allowance (RDA) for sodium. Experts estimate that the body needs about 500 milligrams per day. This is far less than the 4,000 to 6,000 milligrams most Americans get. Most guidelines recommend that daily sodium consumption be limited to 2,400 milligrams or less. This is equal to approximately 6,000 milligrams or one teaspoon of table salt—which is made up of 40 percent sodium and 60 percent chloride.

The Purpose of Sodium

Sodium is an electrolyte that is necessary for good health. It helps maintain fluid balance, helps muscles to contract, is involved in nerve transmissions and helps regulate blood pressure. In terms of food, sodium (salt) is important because it makes food taste better—and taste is the number one reason we choose the foods we eat! Salt is also important as a preservative, and it improves the texture of baked goods and breads.

Lowering Your Salt Intake

Most of the salt in the American diet comes from processed foods, not the salt shaker. Only about 15 percent of the sodium in the average diet is added in the kitchen or at the table. The main sources of salt in the diet include processed meats, prepackaged meals, fast foods, canned and dry soups, cheese, salted snack foods and certain condiments. The best way to learn how much sodium is in a food is to read the label. Foods that provide over 300 milligrams per serving are particularly high in sodium.

UNDERSTANDING THE LABEL

Label	Meaning
Sodium free	Fewer than 5 milligrams of sodium per serving
Very low sodium	35 or fewer milligrams of sodium per serving
Low sodium	140 or fewer milligrams of sodium per serving
Reduced sodium	At least 25 percent less sodium
No added salt	No salt added in processing—does not mean sodium free

In order for a single food item to carry the term "healthy" on the label, it must contain 360 or fewer milligrams per serving. Here's a list of particularly high sources of sodium:

- Canned and dry soups—1 cup = 600-1,300 milligrams
- Cured ham—3 ounces = 1,025 milligrams
- Prepackaged meals (i.e., frozen dinners)—8 ounces = 500-1,570 milligrams
- Processed cheese and cheese spreads—1 ounce = 340-450 milligrams
- Salted popcorn—2 1/2 cups = 330 milligrams
- Soy sauce—1 tablespoon = 1,030 milligrams

While we're born with a preference for sweet tastes, salt is an acquired taste. Many people find that after cutting down on salt, many foods they used to enjoy now taste too salty. Cut down gradually to give your taste buds time to adapt. To consume no more than 2,400 mg/day of sodium, try some of these helpful tips:

- Choose foods that are naturally low in sodium, such as fresh fruits and vegetables.
- Break the habit of adding salt during cooking—there's no reason to salt cooking water—or at the table.
- Rinse canned meats, legumes and vegetables under cold water to remove excess salt.
- Eat a variety of foods during a single meal to stimulate the taste buds.
- Eat meals slowly, savoring the flavor and aroma of each bite.
- You can cut the salt in half or more in most recipes.
- For meals with dried-seasoning packets, use half or less of the packet to cut down on the sodium.
- Learn to season foods with herbs, spices, fruit juice and flavored vinegars.
- Limit processed meats such as ham, bacon, hot dogs and luncheon meats.
- Limit high-salt condiments such as soy sauce, steak sauce, barbecue sauce, mustard and ketchup.
- Buy reduced-salt or low-salt snack foods.
- Watch out for olives, pickles, relishes and many salad dressings.
- When eating out, ask for meals to be prepared with less salt, ask for sauces to be served on the side and avoid using the salt shaker.

HERBS AND SPICES

Using herbs, spices and other flavorings is a great way to make tasty dishes that are low in sodium. You'll have to experiment to find out what works best for you. Here are some tips on using and storing herbs and spices:

- Read the label; some premixed spices contain salt.
- Store herbs and spices in a cool, dark place and in tight containers, avoiding heat, moisture and light.
- Date dry herbs and spices when you buy them; shelf life is about one year.

- Test the freshness of herbs by rubbing them between your fingers and checking the aroma.

- Crumbling dry herbs between your fingers before using releases more flavor.

- Liquid brings out the flavor of dried herbs and spices.

- If you use fresh herbs, store them in a plastic bag in the refrigerator. Before using, wash and pat them dry.

- For soups and stews—dishes that have to cook awhile—add herbs and spices toward the end of cooking.

- For chilled dishes or meats, the earlier you add the herbs and spices, the better the flavor.

- When trying new herbs and spices, add them gradually to the dish. You can always add more.

Seasoning Ideas for Meat and Vegetables

Beef	Bay leaf, dry mustard, marjoram, nutmeg, onion, pepper, sage, thyme
Fish	Curry powder, dill, dry mustard, lemon juice, marjoram, paprika, pepper
Poultry	Ginger, marjoram, oregano, paprika, rosemary, tarragon, sage, thyme
Carrots	Cinnamon, cloves, marjoram, nutmeg, rosemary, sage
Corn	Cumin, curry powder, green pepper, onion, paprika, parsley
Green beans	Dill, curry powder, lemon juice, marjoram, oregano, tarragon, thyme
Peas	Basil, dill, ginger, marjoram, onion, parsley, sage
Potatoes	Basil, dill, garlic, onion, paprika, parsley, rosemary, sage
Squash	Allspice, basil, cinnamon, curry powder, ginger, marjoram, nutmeg, onion, rosemary, sage
Tomatoes	Basil, bay leaf, dill, marjoram, onion, oregano, parsley, pepper, thyme

BUILDING A HEALTHY BODY IMAGE

Pick up any fashion magazine, flip on the TV, and notice the billboards— what do you see? Everywhere we turn, we're presented with unrealistic images of how we should look, what we should wear and how we should live. Beautiful bodies are placed alongside ads for fattening foods, which sends the message that you *can* have it all. How do you measure up to what you see? How do these images and messages influence the way you feel about yourself? Do they influence your lifestyle habits and the goals you set for yourself? Are these messages and ideals in line with God's purpose for your life?

Don't let the media or society's unrealistic expectations influence the goals you set or the way you feel about yourself. Trying to live up to these unrealistic demands will only lead to failure, guilt and disappointment. Set your sight on the more important things in life: your relationship to God, good health and effective living.

Achieving the current ideal body image requires extremes of diet, exercise and cosmetic surgery; it's an image that often comes at the price of good health. Despite what we're led to believe, the ideal body is outside the reach of the majority of men and women and is not a matter of self-discipline. There's absolutely no truth to the prevailing message that thinness equals health and happiness.

WHAT THE NUMBERS SHOW

- Surveys reveal that less than 15 percent of women are happy with their body weight or how they look. Women are three times more likely to be dissatisfied with their appearance than men.
- At any given time nearly 60 percent of women report being on a diet to lose weight; this includes adolescent females. Many women on diets are already at or below a normal body weight.
- Overall, nearly 65 million Americans are dieting at any one time at a cost of over $33 billion dollars each year. Ninety-five percent of people who lose weight gain it all back within five years.

- A decade ago fashion models weighed 8 percent less than the average woman; today they weigh 23 percent less. The average woman is 5'4" and weighs nearly 145 pounds, while the average fashion model is 5'9" and weighs 110 pounds.
- Models and beauty-pageant contestants on average are at least 15 percent below the recommended weight for their height—one of the criteria for diagnosing an eating disorder.
- Eating disorders are on the rise—in both women and men!

Having a positive attitude and accepting who you are is the first step to making healthy lifestyle changes. It often becomes much easier to make permanent lifestyle changes once you accept the reality that you may never have a perfect body shape; the goal now becomes one of good health and better living. Take a moment to consider your reasons for wanting to lose weight.

DETERMINING YOUR SUCCESS

You should primarily judge your success in First Place by how well you meet your goals for good health. Rather than focusing on the scale, set your sights on healthy eating habits and regular physical activity. While you may be able to achieve more, the most successful weight-loss programs result in only a 10- to 15-percent weight loss. That's enough weight loss to improve your health and quality of life but not enough to achieve your ideal body weight. The goal is not to have a perfect figure but to live a healthier, happier and more productive life—in the body that you have! These are goals that everyone can achieve.

There's a popular quote that goes something like this: "Your body is where you'll spend the rest of your life; isn't it about time you made it your home?" Isn't it about time you made it His home too (see 1 Corinthians 6:19-20)?

Do the following exercise with your group. Choose several images or ideas that the media tries to sell. List the messages on the left side of the chart. For each message, decide what God's Word has to say on the matter and list those on the right side of the chart.

What the Media Says	What God Says
Your value is determined by your physical appearance.	*God judges you by your heart (see 1 Samuel 16:7).*

LIFE IN THE
FAST-FOOD LANE

Eating in the fast-food lane has become a way of life for many of us. Life has us on the go, so we often have to eat on the go. Why do people choose to eat fast foods? *Taste, convenience* and *price* top the list. These reasons are important, but good nutrition and health should be at the top of your list.

⟶ Think about why you eat fast food and list your reasons here.

⟶ Do your reasons for eating fast foods influence your ability to make healthy choices? Explain.

FAST-FOOD FARE

What foods do you think of when you think *fast food*: burgers and fries, fried chicken, tacos and burritos, soft drinks? A fast-food meal can easily top 1,000 calories and give you a day's worth of fat, cholesterol and sodium. Believe it or not, you can also make healthy fast-food choices. Today, most fast-food restaurants offer a variety of foods such as grilled chicken, salads, baked potatoes and deli-style sandwiches. Of course, fresh fruits and vegetables are still hard to find. The key is to plan ahead and be prepared to make healthy choices. Look for ways to trim fat, cut calories and add variety whenever you can. Always keep your goals of a healthy weight and good nutrition in mind. Here are some helpful tips; choose the ones that will work best for you.

Eating on the Go

🍎 Order individual items rather than the special meal deal. One item that is higher in calories and fat may be okay, but add fries and a soft drink and you may double the calories and fat.

- Watch out for words like "deluxe," "supersize" or "jumbo." Order the regular or small size instead. A single slice of cheese on a small burger adds calcium. Think nutrition; add the cheese and cut the fries.
- Choose sandwiches with grilled chicken or fish or lean roast beef, turkey or ham. Ask for low-fat toppings like mustard or low-fat salad dressing instead of mayonnaise or special sauce.
- If you're having fast food for one meal, choose healthier foods the rest of the day. Don't forget your fruits and vegetables. You can even carry a piece of fruit with you to eat with your meal.

Lettuce Works

- Beware, salads can have more calories, fat and sodium than a burger and fries! Limit items such as cheese, croutons, bacon, eggs, nuts and creamy salad dressings. Add more vegetables instead.
- Always order salad dressing on the side. Use the low-fat dressing whenever possible. Salsa and low-fat cottage cheese are also good choices. Add flavor with fresh fruits, peppers and other vegetables.
- Limit special salads such as potato, macaroni, tuna and chicken, which are often made with mayonnaise or high-fat salad dressing. More often, choose coleslaw or bean salad made with vinaigrette.

Tater Toppings

- Plain baked potatoes are low in calories and fat, and a good source of fiber and vitamin C. Limit toppings such as butter, cheese, bacon and sour cream.
- Healthier choices include small amounts of margarine and low-fat sour cream. Other good toppings include low-fat cottage cheese, plain yogurt and salsa. Pack on the nutrition by adding lots of fresh vegetables.

Fast-Food Olé

- Choose skinless grilled chicken, beans or vegetables instead of beef or cheese on tostados, tacos or burritos. Ask for your bean burrito to be prepared with less cheese. Order soft tortillas rather than fried.
- Go easy, if at all, on cheese, sour cream and guacamole. Add more lettuce, tomatoes and salsa.

The Orient Express

🍎 Asian takeout is one fast-food option that offers a variety of fresh vegetables. Watch out—portion sizes can be large. Plan to split a dish with a companion or save some for another meal.

🍎 Many dishes include fried meats; ask before you order. Order steamed rice instead of fried rice. Leave off the fried egg roll. Ask for your entreé to be cooked with extra vegetables.

The Pizza Plan

🍎 Pizza can be a healthy choice, but keep these tips in mind: Choose thin crust over thick crust or deep dish and limit yourself to one or two slices.

🍎 Avoid meats such as ground beef and pepperoni that are higher in fat and sodium. Instead, ask for extra tomato sauce and fresh vegetables and less cheese. Order a salad to add variety and nutrition to your meal.

Drink Up

🍎 You can boost the nutrition of any fast-food meal by choosing low-fat milk or natural fruit juices. Remember, water is always a good choice!

🍎 Some milk shakes can equal the calories and fat of an entire meal. Keep this in mind and cut back in other areas if you order the shake.

A Healthy Start

🍎 If breakfast is often a fast-food meal, choose a plain bagel, toast or English muffin with jelly, jam or low-fat cream cheese. Skip the croissant and biscuits, both of which are high in fat and calories.

🍎 Cold or hot cereals with nonfat milk, pancakes without butter or plain scrambled eggs are also good choices. Limit high-fat meats such as bacon and sausage and watch out for fried potatoes.

In the following chart, list the fast-food restaurants you frequent and the foods you usually choose. Next, list some things you can do to make healthier choices. The key is to make a plan and stick with it.

Restaurant	Usual Choices (Be specific)	Better Choices

OUTSMARTING THE SNACK ATTACK

If you want to lose weight, you've got to cut out the snacks! Have you heard this before? It's only partially true. Actually, it's not the snacking that's bad, it's the snacks—high-fat chips and crackers, dips, cookies, candy bars. The truth is that your body works best when it refuels every four to six hours. The best way to fuel your body is to eat light, well-balanced meals and two or three healthy snacks. Snacking may even help you lose weight by "taming" your appetite, thus preventing the tendency to overeat and make poor choices. Learn to make healthy snacks a part of your daily eating plan.

SNACK FACTS

Surveys suggest that 99 percent of Americans snack and 75 percent do so one or more times each day. How much do we spend on snacking? Over $40 million each day. Snacking accounts for nearly 25 percent of daily calories, and by the end of one year the average person has consumed over 22 pounds of snack foods—mostly chips, pretzels, puffs and candy. On the positive side, many of our favorite snack foods now come in low-fat versions. On the down side, many of these are still high in calories and low in nutrition.

➼ Do you snack regularly? What are some of your typical snack foods?

➼ Why do you snack?

☐ To satisfy hunger   ☐ To relax
☐ To satisfy cravings   ☐ For enjoyment and pleasure
☐ To boost energy   ☐ For nourishment
☐ To fight boredom and   ☐ Other_____
    pass time

It's important to understand the reasons why you snack. It's also important to know how your typical snack foods stack up nutritionally. Use snacks to satisfy hunger, nourish your body, boost your energy and help you reach your goals for a healthy weight. Do your snacking habits need an overhaul?

HEALTHY SNACKING

The key to healthy nutrition is variety, balance and moderation. With these principles in mind, snacking can be an important part of a healthy eating plan. Snack time can be a great way to get in your daily servings of fruits, vegetables and whole grains. Low-fat dairy foods such as milk and yogurt also make healthy snacks. Keep a store of healthy snacks with you wherever you are. Concentrate on complex carbohydrates and low-fat proteins. Do whatever you can to avoid those high-fat, high-sugar treats that always seem to show up at home, work and church. Healthy beverages can also be great at snack time—water, fruit or vegetable juice and low-fat milk are your best choices.

When it comes to weight control, the issue is total calories—not when or how often you eat. As for snacking, eat only when you're hungry and stop when you're full!

HOW SNACKS STACK UP

Snack	Calories	Fat (grams)
Ice cream (1 cup)	~ 300	~ 15
Candy bar (2 ounces)	~ 250	~ 12
Mixed nuts (1 ounce or 20 nuts)	~ 200	~ 15
Fried chips (1 ounce or 10 chips)	~ 160	~ 10
Microwave popcorn (3 cups)	~ 150	~ 10
Nonfat fruit yogurt (1 cup)	~ 120	0
Baked chips (1 ounce or 13 chips)	~ 110	~ 1
Pretzels (1 ounce or 9 pretzels)	~ 110	~ 1
Fresh fruit (1 medium)	~ 60	trace
Air-popped popcorn (3 cups)	~ 50	trace
Vegetable (1/2 cup)	~ 25	trace

Plan Ahead

Stock your home, office and workout bag with a variety of healthy snacks, so you'll always have something healthy on hand when hunger strikes. Buy several plastic containers and bags, a thermos and an insulated lunch bag or cooler to make it easy for you to carry snacks with you. Keep a special shopping list to help you remember to stock up on healthy snack foods. Instead of looking for low-fat versions of your favorite processed snack foods, choose foods such as whole-grain breads and crackers, fruits, vegetables, rice cakes and low-fat yogurt, which are all naturally low-fat, low-calorie snacks.

Packable Snacks

animal cookies	low-fat cookies
bagels low-fat	whole-grain crackers
bread sticks	low-fat granola bars
cheese sticks	low-fat popcorn
energy bars	low-fat yogurt
fresh, canned and dried fruits	nonfat chips
fig bars	peanut butter
fruit juice (single-servings)	plain popcorn
graham crackers	precut vegetables
instant oatmeal	pretzels
lean luncheon and canned meats	ready-to-eat cereal
low-fat cheese	water

➤ List some healthy snack ideas you're ready to try.

PUTTING YOUR BEST FOOT FORWARD

In the past, you may have given little thought to the kind of athletic shoes you buy; but if you're going to be serious about a physically active lifestyle, you need to be serious about your feet. Your foot contains 26 bones and has to bear more than six times your body weight during running and jumping activities! A bad pair of shoes can lead to problems as minor as blisters and as major as knee problems.

SELECTING THE RIGHT SHOE

It's important to select the right shoes for your activity. Runners were the first to buy into the idea of specialty shoes, and in 1974 Nike Waffle Trainers became the top-selling athletic shoes. Today experts suggest that people purchase shoes that complement the sport for which they were designed, which means that a person may want several pairs. The following are commonly used:

- **Running**: These are considered forward-motion shoes. They're lightweight, have good cushioning and a raised toe that enables the shoe to roll forward.

- **Walking**: Slightly heavier than some other athletic shoes, they often have features called "roll bars" or "footbridges" that give added support for people who *overpronate* (see definition in next section).

- **Tennis**: These shoes are flatter underneath than a running shoe and, therefore, have more support and stability when moving in a side-to-side or lateral motion. A leather upper gives additional support.

- **Basketball**: Similar to tennis shoes, they have more ankle support and more cushioning for jumping.

- **Cross-trainers**: They're much heavier than running shoes and don't have as much support. They work well for people who enjoy several different activities, but they're not recommended for any one particular sport.

In addition, there are specialty shoes for biking, soccer, hiking and other activities. Seek the advice of someone who really knows your sport before making a purchase.

CHECKING YOUR GAIT

When walking or running, few of us have a neutral gait. Instead, most people roll too far to the inside of the foot, which is called *overpronating*. Others *underpronate* (supinate), meaning that they don't roll enough to the inside. Both gaits can be hard on your feet, knees, hips and back if you have the wrong pair of shoes. Fortunately, a well-fitting shoe can often correct these problems.

What Type of Foot Pattern Do You Have?

Step out of the shower with wet feet and walk across a dry floor. Can you see your entire footprint? If so, you may have a flattened arch and a tendency to overpronate. If you see an island of the forefoot and an island of the heel with dry space between, you probably have a higher arch and a tendency to underpronate. A person who overpronates needs a stiff shoe, whereas someone who underpronates needs a flexible one.

MAKING A PURCHASE

Surprisingly, experts say that about 80 percent of the people are wearing shoes that are too short. It makes sense to take your old pair with you when you shop and to go late in the day when your feet have expanded. Ask a knowledgeable salesperson to evaluate your old shoes, which will help them steer you to the best models. You may want to go to a specialty shop instead of a discount outlet. A good salesperson can look at your shoe and observe several patterns. For example:

> **What do the soles look like?** Where has wear occurred? Many people wear out the outside corner (the point of first contact of the shoe with the ground). Wearing out the inside corner may be a sign of overpronation, which increases your risk of injury if the shoe is not right.

What is the shoe's design? Is the shoe right for the activity you do? Is the shoe comfortable? How does the shoe fit? Is it a special size?

Selecting Brands

There is no one best shoe or brand. Never buy a particular brand or type of shoe just because it works for someone you know. The best shoe is the one that fits your foot. There are several major brands of shoes; most contain the same kinds of rubber, nylon, leather, etc. However, shoes vary from one manufacturer to the next. Try on several pairs, and make your decision based on comfort rather than the brand name.

Buying Tips

- Make sure you have a thumbnail's width of space between your longest toe and the front of the shoe.
- Select shoes based on your weight and foot type. A 100-pound woman, for example, may need a lighter-weight pair of shoes than someone weighing 175 pounds.
- The shoe should be snug without pinching. Don't expect a pair of athletic shoes to fit as tightly as a dress shoe.
- Choose shoes that fit snugly without slipping on your heel.
- Lace up the shoes, and walk, run and jump around the store or outside.
- Remember: If the shoes aren't comfortable in the store, they won't fit well when you get home.
- Sizes vary, depending on the manufacturer. Be willing to try on several sizes until you find the one that fits and feels the best.
- If you find a shoe that works well for you, consider buying a second pair. Models are frequently discontinued. In addition, rotating two pairs helps extend the life of your shoes.
- Don't purchase an ill-fitting pair of shoes just because they're on sale. You may end up paying more in the long run in the form of shin splints, sore knees or other problems.

Replacing Shoes

When to replace shoes depends on how active you are. As a general rule, experts recommend replacing running shoes every 350 to 500 miles. The runner who is heavy and strikes the foot hard against the pavement should replace a shoe closer to the 350-mile range. With a lot of use, you can lose about 60 percent of the cushioning in six months; so even if the shoes don't show major wear, remember that they can quickly lose their shock-absorption capacity and some of their stability. If you start noticing a new ache or pain, it may be time for a new pair of shoes!

Walkers don't need to replace their shoes as often—usually after about 600 miles of use.

Breaking Them In

Of course, it goes without saying that you need to break in a new pair of shoes. Don't purchase running shoes and attempt to run a marathon the next day. Gradually increase the use of a new pair of shoes; it takes a little time for the shoe to form to your foot. By all means, however, use them regularly! With a good pair of shoes, you'll likely get more out of your workout—and your feet will thank you!

QUIET TIME AND PRAYER

In the middle of our busy lives, we often forget that our relationship with God is the foundation from which we grow. The Great Commandment (see Mark 12:28-31) calls us into relationship with Him. Christ is the One for whom you were created (see Colossians 1:15-20), and it is He who gives you strength (see Philippians 4:13). Like any other relationship, however, it takes time and commitment to develop. The time you spend in prayer and in the Word will help you develop intimacy with God and deepen your relationship with Him.

➺ How is your relationship with your heavenly Father?

➺ How much time do you spend in a week talking, listening and sharing your life with the Lord?

➺ In what ways could your quiet time and prayer life be improved?

Prayerfully think about your answers to these questions and begin taking steps to improve your prayer and devotional life. Daily devotions and prayer are lifelines in a hectic world, especially when trying to make lifestyle changes. In the middle of the whirlwind, we can hear Jesus say, "Come away to a quiet place my child, and rest for awhile." He spoke these words to His disciples (see Matthew 11:28); He beckons you to do the same. Your Savior calls you to steal away and spend time with Him. Will you accept His invitation?

Tailoring Your Quiet Times

Having a quiet time is a discipline that must be developed through practice and work. Deep relationships are always intentional. They require time and effort. There are no rules regarding when to do your quiet time; choose what works best for you. Find times and places that will allow you to give the Lord your undivided attention. Perhaps it is in the morning before everyone gets up. It may be in the evening after the children are in bed. Maybe noon is a time when you can get away to be with the Lord.

You also need to learn how you best communicate with Him. Remember that every relationship is unique. Tailor your quiet times to reflect your personal relationship with God. Use the following questions to help you determine the best time, place and ways to devote yourself to quiet time and prayer.

➤ What is your best time of the day for quiet time and prayer? Remember that quality is more important than quantity. Circle one.

Morning   Afternoon   Evening

➤ How much time do you have to spend on devotions? Name a specific time and the amount of time you can spend.

Once you've decided on the best time, write it down on your calendar or in your daily planner in order to establish a routine. Check off each day you successfully keep your date with the Lord. Learn from the days that you don't keep your appointment. Ask yourself what you can do differently next time.

Just as with exercise and other lifestyle changes, many people try to do too much too soon. Set aside an amount of time that works for you. Adjust your schedule as you learn what works best.

Ask friends and family to help you set aside and stick to the times you've set for yourself.

Communing with God

➤ How do you best communicate with God? Check all that apply.

- ☐ Writing
- ☐ Talking
- ☐ Other_____

- ☐ Music
- ☐ Meditating

Take some time to learn how you best communicate and listen to God. It may even be different on different days or at different times of the day. Learn what works best for you. Do you have family and friends with whom you can pray on a regular basis?

➤ Where is your favorite place to meet with God? Check all that apply.

- ☐ Kitchen
- ☐ Outdoors
- ☐ Bedroom
- ☐ Car
- ☐ Other_____

- ☐ Dining Room
- ☐ Office
- ☐ Study
- ☐ Living Room

When you spend time with God, you need to be able to relax and focus your attention. It's important to find a special place where you're comfortable. In Matthew 6:6, Jesus said: "When you pray, go into your room, close the door and pray to your Father, who is unseen. Then your Father, who sees what is done in secret, will reward you."

Studying God's Word

What's your favorite way to study God's Word? There are lots of great ways to study and meditate on God's Word. You need to find what works best for you. Consider the following:

- 🍎 Use a daily devotional as your guide.
- 🍎 Follow a systematic plan for reading through the Bible.
- 🍎 Use a Bible with study notes or other references.
- 🍎 Meditate on and study a favorite verse, passage of Scripture or hymn.

- Get involved in a study group or with an accountability partner and study together. Establish a reading or devotion schedule.
- If you have a long commute to work, listening to the Bible on cassette is an excellent way to spend quality time with the Lord.
- Think of your own creative ideas.

Be prepared before you begin by gathering your materials ahead of time and keep them in a specific place. Or if you like to move around, keep your Bible study materials in a basket, box or other container so that you can pick it up and take it into the next room or outside. In addition to keeping a Bible, notebook and pen or pencil nearby, consider adding a Bible dictionary, other Bible translations, a hymnal or songbook, a journal, a devotional book and anything else you might find helpful. These resources can add variety to your quiet time and having them easily available will encourage you to spend more time studying and praying, rather than looking for them.

USING A PRAYER LIST

You might want to consider developing a prayer list. Keeping and organizing a prayer list can help you focus your prayers on those issues that are most important. When your mind wanders, use your list to get you back on track. Write down the important issues and concerns in your life. Keep an ongoing list of people who need your prayers. Other areas for prayer might include world issues, governmental leaders, missionaries and ministries.

KEEPING PRAYER JOURNALS

Keeping a prayer journal is a great way to keep in touch with God and what's going on in your life. Have you been using the First Place *Prayer Journal* or another tool: notepad, computer, etc.? Keep a record of your prayer requests, answered prayers and other ways God is working in your life and the lives of those around you. As time goes on, you will have a memorial of your journey with Him. Journals help to personalize your devotional time and keep you motivated.

OVERCOMING ROADBLOCKS

Like any discipline, there are obstacles and roadblocks to making quiet time and prayer a part of your daily routine. Do any of these sound familiar?

- *I don't know where to begin.*
- *I don't know how or what to pray.*
- *I don't have time.*
- *I can't seem to keep myself motivated.*
- *The Bible is confusing to me sometimes.*

What are your barriers to quiet time and prayer? How can you overcome them? Talk about your needs and brainstorm solutions with family, friends and your First Place group. Do not forget that quiet time is a discipline to be developed; give yourself time to learn and grow. Even when you don't feel like it, make it a priority to get into the Word and spend some time with your heavenly Father. You'll be glad you did.

FIRST PLACE
MENU PLANS

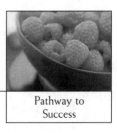

Pathway to
Success

Each plan is based on approximately 1,400 calories.

Breakfast   2 breads, 1 fruit, 1 milk, 0-½ fat
             (When a meat exchange is used, milk is omitted.)

Lunch   2 meats, 2 breads, 1 vegetable, 1 fruit, 1 fat

Dinner   3 meats, 2 breads, 2 vegetables, 1 fat

Snacks   1 bread, 1 fruit, 1 milk, ½-1 fat (or any remaining
             exchanges)

For more calories, add the following to the 1,400-calorie plan.

1,600 calories   2 breads, 1 fat

1,800 calories   2 meats, 3 breads, 1 vegetable, 1 fat

2,000 calories   2 meats, 4 breads, 1 vegetable, 3 fats

2,200 calories   2 meats, 5 breads, 1 vegetable, 1 fruit, 5 fats

2,400 calories   2 meats, 6 breads, 2 vegetables, 1 fruit, 6 fats

The exchanges for these meals were calculated using the MasterCook software. It uses a database of over 6,000 food items prepared using United States Department of Agriculture (USDA) publications and information from food manufacturers. As with any nutritional program, MasterCook calculates the nutritional values of the recipes based on ingredients. Nutrition may vary due to how the food is prepared, where the food comes from, soil content, season, ripeners, processing and methods of preparation. For these reasons, please use the recipes and menu plans as approximate guides. As always, consult your physician and/or a registered dietician before starting a diet program.

Menu Plans for Two Weeks

⬤ Breakfasts

1 c. bran-flakes cereal

1 c. nonfat milk

½ medium papaya

Exchanges: 2 breads, 1 fruit, 1 milk

~~~~~~

2 slices reduced-calorie whole-wheat bread, toasted

1 tbsp. low-fat peanut butter

½ medium grapefruit

1 c. nonfat milk

Exchanges: 1 meat, 1 bread, ½ fruit, 1 fat

~~~~~~

2 low-fat frozen waffles, heated

1 tsp. reduced-calorie margarine

1 tbsp. sugar-free syrup

½ small mango

1 c. nonfat milk

Exchanges: 2 breads, ½ fruit, 1 milk, ½ fat

~~~~~~

Raisin French Toast

1½ slices cinnamon-raisin bread

¼ c. egg substitute

¼ tsp. vanilla flavoring

1 tbsp. nonfat milk

Nonstick cooking spray

In a shallow bowl, combine egg substitute, vanilla and milk; add slices of bread, turning until egg mixture is absorbed. Spray a small nonstick skillet or griddle with nonstick cooking spray; preheat. Cook bread over medium heat 3 to 5 minutes, turning once, until golden brown on both sides.

Serve with 1 tablespoon sugar-free syrup, ½ cup grapefruit sections and ½ cup nonfat milk.

Exchanges: ½ meat, 2 breads, ½ fruit, ½ milk

~~~~~~

1 small (2 oz.) fat-free bran muffin

1 tsp. reduced-calorie margarine

1 tsp. peach jam

½ medium banana

1 c. plain nonfat yogurt

Exchanges: 2 breads, 1 fruit, 1 milk, ½ fat

~~~~~~

1½ c. puffed-wheat cereal

1 large tangerine

1 c. nonfat milk

Exchanges: 2 breads, 1 fruit, 1 milk

~~~~~~

½ large (4 oz.) whole-wheat bagel, toasted

2 tbsp. fat-free cream cheese

1 small orange

1 c. nonfat milk

Exchanges: ½ meat, 2 breads, 1 fruit, 1 milk

~~~~~~

2 frozen low-fat pancakes, heated

1 tbsp. sugar-free syrup

1 tsp. reduced-calorie margarine

2- in. wedge honeydew melon

1 c. nonfat milk

Exchanges: 2 breads, 1 fruit, 1 milk, ½ fat

~~~~~~

1 slice cinnamon-raisin bread, toasted

1 tsp. reduced-calorie margarine

½ tsp. granulated sugar

Pinch cinnamon

¾ c. plain nonfat yogurt

¾ c. blueberries

Exchanges: 1½ breads, 1 fruit, 1 milk, ½ fat

~~~~~~

1 small (2 oz.) whole-wheat English muffin, split and toasted

1 tsp. reduced-calorie margarine

1 c. sliced strawberries

½ c. nonfat milk

Exchanges: 2 breads, 1 fruit, 1 milk, ½ fat

~~~~~~

$\frac{1}{2}$ c. cornflakes cereal

2 slices diet whole-wheat bread, toasted

1 tsp. reduced-calorie margarine

$\frac{1}{2}$ medium banana, sliced

1 c. nonfat milk

Exchanges: 2 breads, 1 fruit, 1 milk, $\frac{1}{2}$ fat

~ ~

3 slices diet sourdough bread, toasted

1 tsp. reduced-calorie margarine

$\frac{3}{4}$ c. blueberries

1 c. nonfat milk

Exchanges: 2 breads, 1 fruit, 1 milk, $\frac{1}{2}$ fat

~ ~

$1\frac{1}{2}$ c. fortified cold cereal

$\frac{1}{2}$ small mango

1 c. nonfat milk

Exchanges: 2 breads, 1 fruit, 1 milk

~ ~

1 small (2 oz.) bagel

1 tsp. strawberry all-fruit spread

$\frac{3}{4}$ c. artificially sweetened mixed-berry nonfat yogurt

$\frac{3}{4}$ c. blackberries

Exchanges: 2 breads, 1 fruit, 1 milk

~ ~

🍎 LUNCH

Chicken and Spinach Salad

2 c. cooked chicken, cubed

6 c. packed fresh spinach
torn into bite-sized pieces

2 oranges, peeled and cut
into chunks

2 c. fresh strawberries, sliced

In large bowl, combine chicken, spinach, oranges and strawberries. Toss with chilled Orange-Poppy Dressing (see following recipe) just before serving. Serves 4.

Serve each with 6 slices melba toast.

Orange-Poppy Dressing

2 tbsp. red wine vinegar	$\frac{1}{4}$ tsp. dry mustard
3 tbsp. orange juice	$\frac{1}{4}$ tsp. poppy seeds
$1\frac{1}{2}$ tbsp. canola oil	

Exchanges: 2 meats, $1\frac{1}{2}$ breads, 1 vegetable, 1 fruit, 1 fat

~~~~~~

Spicy Thai Chicken

2 4-oz. boneless, skinless chicken breasts	$\frac{1}{4}$ tsp. red pepper flakes, crushed
1 small red bell pepper, chopped	1 pkg. artificial sweetener
2 tbsp. white vinegar	1 lime, sliced into 6 wedges

In a food processor, puree red bell pepper with vinegar; pour puree into saucepan. Add red pepper flakes and bring to a boil. Reduce heat; simmer 3 minutes. Remove from heat. Once cooled, stir in artificial sweetener.

Broil chicken breasts in preheated oven 10 minutes or until browned. Once browned, turn pieces and broil approximately 5 minutes more.

While broiling chicken, prepare serving platter with a bed of hot cooked white or brown rice, or couscous. Remove chicken from oven and place on bed of rice/couscous. Spoon sauce over chicken; garnish with lime wedges and serve immediately. Serves 2.

Serve each with $\frac{2}{3}$ cup rice (or couscous) and $\frac{1}{2}$ cup sautéed snap peas.
Exchanges: 2 lean meat, 2 breads, 1 vegetable, $\frac{1}{2}$ fat

~~~~~~

Shrimp Cocktail

4 iceberg lettuce leaves
$2\frac{1}{2}$ oz. medium shrimp, cooked, peeled and deveined
1 tbsp. cocktail sauce
3 slices (1 oz. total) pumpernickel bread

Line plate with lettuce leaves; top with shrimp and cocktail sauce.

Serve with Pickled Beet and Onion Salad (see following recipe) and 1 medium kiwi fruit.

Pickled Beet and Onion Salad

1 c. cooked, sliced beets
½ c. onion, sliced
2 tbsp. cider vinegar
Freshly ground pepper,
to taste

1 tsp. canola oil
Sugar substitute to equal
2 tsp. sugar

In a medium bowl, combine beets, onion, cider vinegar, canola oil, sugar substitute and ground pepper to taste. Refrigerate covered at least 1 hour.
Exchanges: 2 meats, 1 bread, 2 vegetables, 1 fruit, 1 fat

~~~~~~

Sliced-Egg Sandwich

2 slices diet whole-wheat bread
1 hard-boiled egg, sliced
¼ c. watercress leaves

2 tomato slices
2 tsp. low-fat mayonnaise

Serve with ½ cup each carrot and celery sticks and a 3x2-inch wedge of watermelon.
Exchanges: 1 meat, 1 bread, 1 vegetable, 1 fruit, 1 fat

~~~~~~

Skinless Roast Chicken Breast

2 oz. boneless, skinless roasted chicken breast
⅔ c. wide noodles (cooked with 1 tsp. reduced-calorie margarine)
1 c. cooked, sliced beets

Serve with Spinach Salad (see following recipe) and ¾ cup plain nonfat yogurt mixed with ½ cup drained canned peach slices (no sugar added).

Spinach Salad

2 c. spinach leaves, torn
½ c. mushrooms, sliced
½ c. red onion

1 tbsp. imitation bacon bits
1 tbsp. fresh lemon juice

Exchanges: 2 meats, 2 breads, 2 vegetables, 1 fruit, 1 milk, ½ fat

~~~~~~

Grilled Turkey Burger

2 oz. grilled ground turkey
1 slice nonfat processed
   American cheese
2 oz. hamburger roll

1 c. tomato
1 c. Spanish onion slices
2 iceberg lettuce leaves

Serve with Russian Dressing and Oven Fries (see following recipes).

Russian Dressing

In small cup or bowl, combine $2\frac{1}{2}$ teaspoons each low-fat mayonnaise and ketchup.

Oven Fries

1 3-oz. baking potato,
   cut into thin sticks
$\frac{1}{4}$ tsp. salt

$\frac{1}{4}$ tsp. paprika
   Nonstick cooking spray

Preheat oven to 450° F. Place potato sticks onto nonstick baking sheet; spray sticks lightly with nonstick cooking spray. Sprinkle with salt and paprika; bake 10 to 12 minutes or until crispy outside and tender inside.
Exchanges: $2\frac{1}{2}$ meats, 3 breads, 1 vegetable, 1 fat

~~~~~~

2 oz. baked lean ham
3 oz. baked sweet potato
1 tsp. reduced-calorie margarine
1 c. combined steamed sliced zucchini and yellow squash

Serve with Cucumber and Tomato Salad drizzled with Balsamic Vinaigrette (see following recipes), a 1-ounce dinner roll and 1 teaspoon reduced calorie margarine.

Cucumber and Tomato Salad

1 medium tomato
$\frac{1}{2}$ cucumber

Balsamic Vinaigrette

2 tsp. balsamic vinegar
1 tsp. olive oil
   Pinch garlic powder

Quarter tomato and cucumber; place in small salad bowl. Combine vinegar, olive oil and garlic powder in small jar with tight-fitting lid; cover and shake well. (Can also be made in small bowl and blended with wisk.) Pour over cucumbers and tomatoes.

Exchanges: 2 meats, 2 breads, 2 vegetables, 1 fat

~~~~~~

2 oz. boneless grilled pork chop

⅔ c. cooked brown rice

1 tsp. reduced-calorie margarine

½ tsp. caraway seeds

1 c. steamed cabbage

Serve with 1 cup tossed green salad and 2 tablespoons fat-free ranch dressing.

Exchanges: 2 meats, 2 breads, 2 vegetables, 1 fruit, 1 fat

~~~~~~

2 oz. roasted turkey

⅔ c. roasted new potatoes

1 c. steamed cauliflower

¾ c. blueberries

Serve with 2 cups Bibb lettuce tossed with ½ cup radish, ¼ cup croutons and 2 tablespoons balsamic vinegar.

Exchanges: 2 meats, 2 breads, 1 vegetable, 1 fruit

~~~~~~

Stuffed Sweet Potato

1 6-oz. baked sweet potato

2 oz. lean ham, diced

1 tsp. reduced-fat margarine

1 tbsp. raisins

Dash cinnamon

Serve with 1 cup steamed asparagus spears drizzled with 1 tablespoon Balsamic Vinaigrette (see recipe on page 191).

Exchanges: 2 meats, 2 breads, 2 vegetables, ½ fruit, 1 fat

~~~~~~

Chicken Fajita

1 ½ oz. cooked chicken, shredded
¼ c. onion, diced
¼ c. bell pepper, diced
¼ c. salsa

1 tbsp. fat-free sour cream
1 10-in. low-fat flour tortilla
¼ oz. Colby cheese, shredded
Nonstick cooking spray

In skillet coated with cooking spray, sauté onion and pepper for 1 minute; add chicken and heat thoroughly. In small bowl, combine salsa and sour cream; mix well. Fill tortilla with chicken; top with cheese. Heat in microwave, if desired, and serve with creamy salsa.

Serve with 1 cup canned tropical mixed fruit.

Exchanges: 2 meats, 2 breads, 1 ½ vegetables, 1 fruit, 1 fat

~~~~~~

Grilled Turkey and Cheese Sandwich

1 ½-oz. slice cooked turkey breast
2 slices whole-wheat diet bread
1 tsp. low-fat mayonnaise

1 tsp. mustard
½-oz. slice Swiss cheese
Butter-flavored nonstick cooking spray

Preheat skillet; coat with cooking spray. Spread mayonnaise and mustard on bread; layer with turkey and cheese. Grill sandwich over medium heat until bread is lightly browned on both sides and cheese is melted, turning occasionally.

Serve with Cucumber and Tomato Salad drizzled with 1 tablespoon Balsamic Vinaigrette (see recipes on page 191) and 1 ounce reduced-fat pretzels.

Exchanges: 2 meats, 2 breads, 1 vegetable, 1 fat

~~~~~~

Captain D's or Long John Silver's Baked Fish Dinner

½ c. rice
½ c. steamed or grilled vegetables
2 hush puppies or 1 small (1 oz.) breadstick

Exchanges: 3 meats, 2 breads, 1 vegetable, 1 fat

~~~~~~

Arby's Junior Roast Beef Sandwich

1 c. green salad
2 tbsp. low-fat salad dressing
1 banana

Exchanges: 2 meats, 2 breads, 1 vegetable, 1 fruit, 1 fat

~~~~~~

🍎 DINNER

BBQ Steak Kabobs

$1\frac{1}{4}$-lbs. boneless round- or top-sirloin
    steaks, cut into 2-in. pieces
2 tbsp. plus 2 tsp. ketchup
1 tbsp. light molasses
1 tbsp. plus 1 tsp. Worcestershire
    sauce

2 tsp. spicy brown mustard
2 tsp. grated onion
4 slices French bread, cut $\frac{1}{2}$ in.
    thick, toasted and hot
1 garlic clove, halved

Preheat grill to medium. In large bowl, combine ketchup, molasses, Worcestershire, mustard and onion; season with salt to taste. Add meat; toss to coat well. Thread steak chunks onto long skewers; grill to desired doneness (10 minutes for medium rare) turning occasionally and brushing with sauce. While skewers are cooking, toast French bread. Lightly rub one side of hot toasted bread with cut side of garlic clove. Serves 4.

    Serve each with 1 cup grilled vegetables and $\frac{1}{2}$ cup roasted potatoes.
Exchanges: 3 meats, 2 breads, 2 vegetables, 1 fat

~~~~~~

Tuna and Broccoli Casserole

6 oz. cooked elbow macaroni,
    rinsed and drained
3 c. frozen broccoli, thawed
1 9-oz. can white tuna, packed in
    water, drained and flaked
1 8-oz. can sliced water chestnuts,
    drained
$\frac{3}{4}$ c. (or 3 oz.) shredded reduced-
    fat cheddar cheese

1 $10\frac{3}{4}$ oz. can reduced-fat
    cream of mushroom soup
1 c. plain nonfat yogurt
$\frac{1}{3}$ c. dry nonfat milk powder
1 tsp. cornstarch
1 tsp. Worcestershire sauce
$\frac{1}{2}$ tsp. granulated garlic
$\frac{1}{4}$ c. Parmesan cheese, grated
    Butter flavored nonstick
    cooking spray

Preheat oven to 350° F. Spray 8x8-inch cooking dish with cooking spray. In a large bowl, combine macaroni, broccoli, tuna, water chestnuts and cheddar cheese. In separate bowl, combine soup, yogurt, milk powder, cornstarch, Worcestershire sauce and garlic. Blend well. Add soup mixture to macaroni mixture; mix well to combine. Pour into prepared casserole. Sprinkle with Parmesan. Cover and bake for 30 minutes. Uncover and bake an additional 10 minutes. Serves 4.

Serve each with 1 cup green salad and 2 tablespoons low-fat dressing.
Exchanges: 2 meats, 2½ breads, 1 vegetable, ½ milk, 1½ fats

~~~~~~

BBQ Chicken Breasts with Apricot Glaze

4 chicken breast halves (about 1½ lbs.), skin on and bone in

⅓ c. apricot preserves　　　　　2 tbsp. plus 2 tsp. ketchup

1 tbsp. soy sauce　　　　　　　　2 tsp. brown sugar

1 tbsp. water

Preheat grill to medium. Grill chicken (skin on) 10 minutes, turning occasionally. Remove from grill and remove skin. In small bowl, combine preserves, soy sauce, water, ketchup and brown sugar; blend well. Return chicken to grill; generously brush with glaze. Continue cooking 10 to 15 minutes or until thoroughly done, turning often and brushing with glaze frequently. Serves 4.

Serve each with 1 cup mashed potatoes and 1 cup seasoned green beans.
Exchanges: 3 meats, 2 breads, 2 vegetables, 1 fat

~~~~~~

Crock-Pot Chicken Stew

2 c. water

4 4-oz. boneless, skinless chicken breasts, cut into chunks

1 16-oz. can navy beans, drained

1 16-oz. can low-sodium stewed tomatoes

½ c. thinly sliced celery

1½ c. diced carrot

½ c. chopped onion

⅛ tsp. garlic powder

1 bay leaf

½ tsp. crushed dry leaf basil

¼ tsp. crushed dry leaf oregano

¼ tsp. paprika

1 tsp. low-sodium instant chicken or beef boullion

Combine all ingredients in Crock-Pot; cook on low heat 8 to 10 hours. Discard bay leaf before serving. Serves 4.

Serve each with a 2-inch cube of cornbread.

Exchanges: 3 meats, 2 breads, 2 vegetables, 1 fat

~~~~~~

Citrus-Braised Chicken Breasts with Capers

4 4-oz. boneless, skinless chicken breasts
3 garlic cloves, minced
1 small onion, thinly sliced
½ tsp. ground cumin
½ c. orange juice
1 tbsp. lemon juice
1 tsp. orange peel, grated (orange part only)
¼ tsp. ground pepper
2 tsp. capers
Olive oil nonstick cooking spray

Rinse chicken and pat dry. Preheat nonstick skillet sprayed with cooking spray. Brown chicken on both sides over medium-high heat; remove from pan. Reduce heat and recoat pan with cooking spray. Add garlic; stir until browned slightly. Add onion; continue cooking, stirring until onion begins to brown. Stir in cumin, citrus juices, orange peel and pepper. Add chicken; cover and simmer for 10 minutes. Add capers and simmer covered 5 to 8 minutes or until chicken is tender.

Top each breast with onions, capers and 1 tablespoon citrus sauce prior to serving. Serves 4.

Serve each with ⅔ cup cooked rice and 1 cup sautéed snap peas.

Exchanges: 3 meats, 2 breads, 1 vegetable, ½ fat

~~~~~~

10- to 11-Ounce Frozen Dinner Entrée with Meat

Serve with spinach salad with mandarin oranges and reduced-fat sweet and sour dressing, and 1 toasted breadstick spread with 1 teaspoon reduced-fat margarine.

Exchanges: 2 meats, 2 breads, 1 vegetable, ½ fruit, 1 fat

~~~~~~

Ginger and Garlic Braised Halibut Fillets

1¼ lbs. 1-in. thick halibut fillets, cut into 4 pieces
1 small onion, minced
2 white scallions, chopped
2 green scallions, chopped into 1-in. lengths
3 garlic cloves, minced
2 tbsp. minced fresh ginger
⅛ tsp. red pepper flakes, crushed
¼ c. white grape juice
½ c. canned chicken broth
2 c. instant brown rice, uncooked
Nonstick cooking spray

Lightly coat large nonstick skillet with cooking spray. Preheat until very hot but not smoking. Add fillets; brown skin side down for 2 minutes. Add onion, scallions, garlic, ginger and red pepper flakes; cook on high 1 minute. Reduce heat; turn fillets. Add grape juice and broth; cover pan and simmer 10 minutes or until cooked through. (Insert small, thin knife into fish to check for doneness.)

While fish is simmering, prepare 4 servings instant brown rice according to package directions. Serve fish over rice and spoon some of the sauce over the fillets. Serves 4.

Serve each with 1 cup Broccoli Slaw (see following recipe) and ⅔ cup rice.

Broccoli Slaw

1 16-oz. bag shredded broccoli slaw mix
¼ c. sweet pickle relish
⅓ c. low-fat mayonnaise
1 tsp. prepared brown mustard
¼ tsp. celery seed
¼ tsp. black pepper
1 c. (about 15) red grapes (optional)

Combine all ingredients in large bowl; refrigerate until needed. Serves 4.
Exchanges: 3 meats, 2 breads, 2 vegetables, 1 fat

~~~~~~

Grilled Swordfish with Oregano

2 8-oz. swordfish steaks
1 garlic clove, crushed
¼ tsp. dill weed, divided
½ tsp. dried leaf oregano, divided
Nonstick cooking spray
¼ c. lemon juice
⅛ tsp. paprika (or to taste)
Salt to taste (added during (cooking)

Preheat grill or broiler to medium-high heat. Rub steaks with garlic; place on hot grill or broiler pan coated with cooking spray. Sprinkle with half the dill, half the oregano and a little salt. Cook 4 to 5 minutes; turn and brush with lemon juice. Season with remaining dill and oregano, and a little more salt. Cook additional 4 to 5 minutes or until fish is opaque throughout. Cut each in half; sprinkle with paprika. Serves 4.

Serve each with 1 twice-baked potato and 1 cup sautéed spinach.
Exchanges: 3 meats, 2 breads, 2 vegetables, 1 fat

~ ~

Chicken Breasts with Asparagus and Carrots

4 4-oz. boneless, skinless chicken breasts, cut crosswise into $\frac{1}{4}$-in. strips	1 small onion, thinly sliced
$\frac{1}{2}$ lb. fresh asparagus spears, trimmed and cut into 1-in. lengths	2 tbsp. reduced-fat margarine, melted
2 medium carrots, cut into $\frac{1}{8}$ in. thick rounds	2 tsp. lemon juice
	$\frac{1}{2}$ tsp. tarragon
	$\frac{1}{8}$ tsp. cayenne pepper
	Salt and pepper to taste

Preheat oven to 450° F. Tear off a large piece of aluminum foil for each serving. Arrange chicken in center of lower half of each length of foil. Season with salt and pepper; top with equal amounts of asparagus, carrot and onion. In small bowl, combine melted margarine, lemon juice, tarragon and cayenne pepper; salt to taste. Pour equal amounts of liquid over each serving of chicken. For each serving, fold two ends of foil together and tightly fold three or four times. Repeat process with ends to seal packet tightly. Arrange foil packets in a single layer on baking sheet; bake 20 minutes and serve. Serves 4.

Serve each with a 1-ounce dinner roll and $\frac{1}{2}$ cup cooked rice.
Exchanges: 3 meats, 2 breads, 1 vegetable, 1 fat

~ ~

Chicken Cacciatore Pie

1 lb. ground chicken breast

1 15-oz. can Italian-style diced tomatoes, drained (reserve 3½ tbsp. juice)

¾ small onion, chopped

¾ small green bell pepper, chopped

1 garlic clove, minced

⅓ c. plain bread crumbs

1 egg

1¼ tsp. Italian herb seasoning

⅓ c. fat-free mozzarella cheese, shredded

2 tbsp. Parmesan cheese, grated

Preheat oven to 350° F. In medium bowl, combine reserved tomato juice, onion, bell pepper, garlic, bread crumbs and egg. Add half the Italian seasoning; salt and pepper to taste. Mix thoroughly. Add ground chicken; mix well. Pat mixture evenly into lightly oiled 10-inch pie plate, pushing up sides to form a shell. Bake 25 minutes.

In stainless steel saucepan, combine tomatoes and remaining Italian seasoning; salt and pepper to taste. Simmer 10 to 15 minutes over medium heat; remove from heat and set aside. Remove meat shell from oven; discard excess liquid. Sprinkle shell with mozzarella cheese. Add tomato sauce, sprinkle with Parmesan cheese and bake 15 minutes until meat shell is cooked throughout. Let stand 5 minutes before cutting and serving. Serves 4.

Serve each with 1 cup green salad, 2 tablespoons low-fat dressing and a 1-ounce slice toasted French bread.

Exchanges: 3 meats, 2 breads, 2 vegetables, 2 fats

~ ~

Chicken and Green Bean Dinner

2½ lbs. skinless chicken pieces, bone in

1 tbsp. all-purpose flour

1 11-oz. can reduced-fat cream of mushroom soup

1 10-oz. pkg. frozen green beans, thawed

½ c. chicken broth

⅛ tsp. paprika

¾ lb. potatoes, scrubbed and cut into 2-in. pieces

Salt and pepper to taste

Preheat oven to 350° F. Place flour in oven-roasting bag. Add soup, green beans and chicken broth to flour; salt and pepper to taste. Squeeze bag to blend mixture. Place bag in baking pan and arrange ingredients in an even layer in bag. Sprinkle chicken with paprika; add salt and pepper. Place chicken and potatoes inside roasting bag on top of green bean mixture. Close bag and cut 4 ½-inch slits in top. Bake 45 to 50 minutes or until chicken is tender. Serves 4.

Serve each with 1 cup Broccoli Slaw (see recipe on page 197) and a 1-ounce dinner roll.

Exchanges: 3 meats, 2 breads, 2 vegetables, 1 ½ fats

~~~~~~

Seafood Restaurant Dinner

Broiled or grilled seafood restaurant seafood entrée (lunch-sized portion, sauce on the side)

½ c. rice
½ c. steamed or grilled vegetables
2 c. salad
2 tbsp. low-fat dressing (on the side)

Exchanges: 3 meats, 2 breads, 2 vegetables, 2 fats

~~~~~~

Spaghetti Carbonara

6 oz. uncooked spaghetti noodles
1 tsp. vegetable oil
1 medium onion, chopped
⅔ c. reduced-sodium chicken broth
3 c. sliced mushrooms
8 oz. lean Canadian bacon, thinly sliced into strips

1 c. frozen peas
1 oz. freshly grated Parmesan cheese
2 tbsp. reduced-fat sour cream
Freshly ground black pepper
Additional Parmesan cheese for garnish (optional)
Nonstick cooking spray

Cook spaghetti noodles according to package directions, omitting salt and fat; drain. Return to pot; toss with oil to prevent sticking. Set aside. Coat large, nonstick skillet with cooking spray. Sauté onion over medium-high heat until tender. Add broth; bring to a boil. Add mushrooms; cook 4 to 5 minutes, stirring frequently. Add bacon strips. Cook additional 2 to 3 minutes; add peas. When heated through, remove from heat. Stir in cheese and sour cream. Garnish each serving with pepper and fresh Parmesan. Serves 4.

Serve each with 1 cup green salad, 2 tablespoons low-fat dressing and a 1-ounce slice of toasted French bread.

Exchanges: 2 ½ meats, 2 ½ breads, 1 vegetable, 1 fat

~~~~~~

Southwestern Snapper

1½ lbs. snapper fillets,
  cut into 4 6-oz. portions
¼ c. lime juice
½ c. egg substitute
1 c. finely crushed ranch-flavored
  tortilla chips

1 c. chunky salsa
¼ c. chopped fresh cilantro
Nonstick cooking spray

Preheat oven to 450° F. Rinse fillets with cold water and pat dry with paper towels. Combine lime juice and egg substitute in shallow dish. Place tortilla crumbs in separate dish. Dip each fillet into egg mixture; press into seasoned crumbs to coat. Place on baking sheet coated with cooking spray and sprinkle with any remaining crumbs. Bake 10 to 12 minutes or until fish flakes with fork. Top each fillet with ¼ cup salsa and garnish with cilantro. Serves 4.

Serve each with 1 cup Broccoli Slaw (see recipe on page 197) and ½ cup garlic mashed potatoes.

Exchanges: 3 meats, 2 breads, 1 vegetable, 1 fat

CONVERSION CHART
EQUIVALENT IMPERIAL AND METRIC MEASUREMENTS

Liquid Measures

Fluid Ounces	U.S.	Imperial	Milliliters
	1 teaspoon	1 teaspoon	5
¼	2 teaspoons	1 dessert spoon	7
½	1 tablespoon	1 tablespoon	15
1	2 tablespoons	2 tablespoons	28
2	¼ cup	4 tablespoons	56
4	½ cup or ¼ pint		110
5		¼ pint or 1 gill	140
6	¾ cup		170
8	1 cup or ½ pint		225
9			250 or ¼ liter
10	1¼ cups	½ pint	280
12	1½ cups or ¾ pint		340
15		3/4 pint	420
16	2 cups or 1 pint		450
18	2¼ cups		500 or ½ liter
20	2½ cups	1 pint	560
24	3 cups or 1½ pints		675
25		1¼	700
30	3¾ cups	1½ pints	840
32	4 cups		900
36	4½ cups		1000 or 1 liter
40	5 cups	2 pints or 1 quart	1120
48	6 cups or 3 pints		1350
50		2½ pints	1400

Solid Measures

U.S. and Imperial Measures		Metric Measures	
Ounces	Pounds	Grams	Kilos
1		28	
2		56	
3½		100	
4	¼	112	
5		140	
6		168	
8	½	225	
9		250	¼
12	¾	340	
16	1	450	
18		500	½
20	1¼	560	
24		675	
27		750	¾
32	2	900	
36	2¼	1000	1
40	2½	1100	
48	3	1350	
54		1500	1½
64	4	1800	
72	4½	2000	2
80	5	2250	2¼
100	6	2800	2¾

Oven Temperature Equivalents

Fahrenheit	Celsius	Gas Mark	Description
225	110	$\frac{1}{4}$	Cool
250	130	$\frac{1}{2}$	
275	140	1	Very Slow
300	150	2	
325	170	3	Slow
350	180	4	Moderate
375	190	5	
400	200	6	Moderately Hot
425	220	7	Fairly Hot
450	230	8	Hot
475	240	9	Very Hot
500	250	10	Extremely Hot

LEADER'S DISCUSSION GUIDE

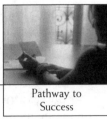

Week One: Dream of Success

1. Discuss the quote, "Success is the progressive realization of a worthwhile dream." Lead group members to give examples, i.e., completing college, paying off a debt or buying a house. Summarize: Success is each step along the pathway to our dreams. A pathway is the route or course we follow. Our pathway is not uncharted territory. Our Savior has walked the pathway to success. We must follow His footsteps. Read 1 Peter 2:21.

2. Call on a volunteer to read Jeremiah 33:3. Form groups of three or four and then ask members to share the dreams they identified in Day 1. Remind members that sharing is voluntary. This would be a good opportunity to remind members about the confidentiality of things shared with the group.

3. Reconvene the whole group. Using a white or chalkboard or newsprint, develop the group's definition of success. Invite members to look at their notes from Day 2. Contrast this definition with the world's view of success. Discuss: What are some of the conditions needed for success in First Place? Write responses beneath the definition.

4. Point out that not all of our dreams are realized, and many others may not be fulfilled for a number of years. From your own experience, share a shattered dream that has been restored or perhaps replaced with a new dream. Call for other testimonies from volunteers. Relate the concept of shattered and restored dreams to weight-loss or other health issues. Review the five truths at the conclusion of Day 3 (p. 14).

5. From Day 4 review the concept that pleasing ourselves or pleasing others will not be a sufficient motivation for most of us to stay with the First Place program. Discuss: What is a more sufficient motivation? (Pleasing God.) Call on volunteers to share why they have chosen to be a part of this group.

6. Discuss: How does seeking the heart of God help us make choices and determine priorities? Ask someone to recall why this program is called First Place. Refer to Matthew 6:33.

7. Discuss: How can sharing your dreams with your First Place group help you accomplish them? After several responses, discuss: What are the risks in sharing our dreams? (Having to be accountable, embarrassment if we do not achieve goals.) Encourage members to risk vulnerability with each other.

   Discuss the concept of praying the Scriptures from Day 6. Encourage members to begin to include praying the Scriptures in their personal prayer time.

8. If time allows, discuss the quote by Martin Luther King, Jr., from Day 7. Discuss the importance of pursuing dreams and goals even though there may be difficulties to face. Encourage members to include in their dreams and goals the vision of a more intimate relationship with Christ.

9. Review the Scripture memory verse. Close with prayer, using one of the Scripture prayers from Day 6 or 7.

Week Two: Plan for Success

1. Bring a set of blueprints, if possible. Discuss their purpose. Ask if anyone has been involved in building a new house. Let him or her share experiences with developing plans for the house. Conclude by explaining: God has a master plan for our lives uniquely fitted to us according to His design.

2. Have the group read Jeremiah 29:11 in unison. Ask for a definition of the word "prosper." Read John 10:10. Discuss how the word "prosper" appropriately describes God's plan for us. Help them understand that prosperity can mean more than material or monetary success.

3. Discuss: Why is trusting God's plans sometimes difficult? Do you ever have fears about what God's plans might mean for you or a loved one? Invite volunteers to share why they consider God to be trustworthy.

4. Lead a discussion of Luke 14:26-33 from Day 2. Using the board to record responses, brainstorm the sacrifices that we may need to make as a part of First Place. Conclude the discussion by asking: What is the cost of not following God's plan? Then have a volunteer read Colossians 3:1.

5. Call on someone to share a long-range goal that requires several short-range goals to achieve it. Write the long-range goal on the board, and lead the group to brainstorm the short-range goals that

would be necessary to complete it. Encourage members to follow this procedure for each of the goals they identified in Day 1 of week one. If time permits, use this procedure to work through a second long-range goal.

6. From Day 4, discuss the need to manage our time. Ask members how they responded to the questions about changes that might be needed in how they use time. Develop a group answer to the question: What should be your priority in the use of your time? Discuss the struggle inherent in the demands on our time.

7. Invite a volunteer to review how being flexible about their priorities kept Paul and Silas focused on God's plan for them (see Acts 16:16-34). Share a personal experience or ask for a volunteer to share about a time when God had another plan than the one expected and how that experience worked out. Before concluding the meeting, ask several members to recite this week's Scripture memory verse.

8. Discuss the SMART and WISE goals (pp. 34-35). Preface discussion by saying everyone can participate, even if they did not read Days 6 and 7. Write the acrostics on the board and discuss each point.

9. Lead in prayer asking God for willingness to listen to Him daily for instructions and guidance.

Week Three: Surrender for Success

1. **Before the meeting**, research the dictionary definitions of the words "surrender" and "wholehearted" and bring them to the session. Or ask members to bring the definitions when you contact them during the week. Write the five days' titles for this week's lessons on a poster board for display during the session.

2. Recite this week's Scripture memory verse together to begin the session. Share the definitions of the words "surrender" and "wholehearted." Or have the members share their definitions. Compose a group statement of what it means to wholeheartedly surrender to God. Write the statement on the board.

3. Display the poster listing the seven areas we are to surrender to God. Have members form groups of two or three. Assign one of the areas to each small group. If you have fewer than seven groups, assign the areas you feel are most pertinent to your members. Be prepared to speak to the unassigned areas yourself during the reporting session.

Give the following small-group assignment: Describe the attitudes and actions of a person who has surrendered this area of his or her life to God.

After a few minutes of discussion, call for the small-group reports. After each report, use the following supplemental discussion questions before moving on to the next area. Watch the time so that each group will be able to report. If necessary, give your report on the areas that were unassigned.

- Day 1: How does Jesus help us take off the old self and put on the new self?
- Day 1: How have you found Jesus sufficient as your Bread of Life?
- Day 2: What should be our attitude in serving Christ?
- Day 3: How do attitudes impact our actions and vice versa?
- Day 4: How does faith help us to be Christ-controlled and not fear-controlled?
- Day 4: Why do we tend to trust our wisdom rather than God's?
- Day 5: How can getting your body in the best shape be an act of worship?

4. If time allows, discuss the questions in Day 6 regarding surrender and behavior. Then discuss the difference between giving up or giving in and giving over. Discuss how to surrender as presented on Day 7.

5. Close the meeting by asking two or three members to read one of the Scripture prayers before you say a final prayer.

Week Four: Dress for Success

1. Discuss the importance of dressing for success in the business and professional world. Discuss the parallel point that Christians need to dress for success in order to protect themselves from Satan. Recite this week's Scripture memory verse together.

2. Note that the armor of God is not automatically on our bodies when we wake up in the morning. Putting on our armor requires action on our part. Discuss actions that are necessary to put on the full armor: prayer, Bible study, Scripture memorization, worship, daily lifestyle choices.

3. **Before the meeting,** obtain a picture of a soldier in full armor. Display the picture at this point. List the pieces of armor named in Ephesians 6:10-17 on the left-hand side of the board as members call them out. Have members explain the purpose of each piece of armor and write the purpose beside each one.

4. Give members an opportunity to study the chart they have helped complete. Discuss: Which piece of armor is unnecessary? Which piece could be left off and yet still allow the soldier to be successful in battle?

5. Point out that battle armor is pointless unless you know the enemy you are fighting. Read 1 Peter 5:8. Discuss: What is the devil's purpose? (To destroy us.) Read John 8:44. Continue: What is one of Satan's most effective strategies? (Lies.) What are some other enemies we might encounter? (Ourselves, our fleshly nature and others.) Discuss the old saying "I am my own worst enemy."

6. Discuss ways that Christians cooperate with, rather than fight against, Satan. Form groups of two to three. Instruct small groups to take prayer requests for ways that members have experienced Satan's interference in their own lives. Remind the group of the need for confidentiality and affirm that sharing is voluntary. Observe groups as they discuss, offering help when needed. Reconvene the whole group when most are finished praying.

7. Read Ephesians 6:18. Discuss the need to stay alert and the role prayer has in keeping us alert. Note that Paul encouraged us to pray for each other. Tell how much you appreciate the members' prayers for you. Allow prayer testimonies as time permits. Share from your own life or ask a volunteer to share about how prayer and God's Word have served as weapons in his or her life to defeat a difficult enemy.

8. From Day 7 discuss self-control. Pray for anyone who may feel like they are out of control.

9. After prayer time, close the session by singing a familiar hymn about prayer, or play a recorded song that you feel would encourage members to turn to Jesus for victory in their everyday battles with Satan.

Week Five: Keys to Success

1. **Before the meeting,** draw the outline of a key (make it as large as possible) on seven pieces of construction paper or poster board and

cut them out. List the following seven pairs of words on the keys (one pair on each key): "Commitment and Effort," "Obedience and Blessings," "Honesty and Integrity," "Wisdom and Understanding," "Courage and Strength," "Support and Encouragement" and "Patience and Fortitude." Prepare to display these as you discuss each key to success.

2. As the meeting begins, have members take their keys out of their purse or pocket and share what kinds of keys they have on their key rings. Ask what other keys they keep at home, such as keys to boats, storage buildings and so forth. Point out that the purpose of keys is to unlock what we otherwise would not be able to enter. Explain: Jesus is the key to heaven and the key to abundant life here on Earth. He is also the key to locking out the power of sin and Satan.

3. Recite this week's Scripture memory verse in unison. Have members offer sentence paraphrases of the verse.

4. Display the first key on the wall or board. Discuss: What is the relationship between commitment and effort? Invite volunteers to share commitments they checked and the efforts they will take to keep those commitments.

5. Display the second key. Ask: What are some blessings of obedience in the First Place program? What are some consequences of disobedience?

6. Display the third key. Discuss the impact of honesty and integrity on success in the First Place program. Discuss weighing and measuring foods accurately and being honest with oneself and with God.

7. Display the fourth key. Discuss the differences between a wise person and a fool, based on the Proverbs passages. Then have members name sources of wisdom and understanding, i.e., prayer, Bible study, Christian friends, church staff, worship, sermons, music, appropriate godly books and magazines.

8. Display the fifth key of courage and strength. Share a fear or anxiety that God has helped you overcome. Allow volunteers to share any fears they might have about failing the First Place program.

9. As you support and encourage them, display the sixth key. Encourage testimonies of how group members have ministered to one another.

10. Display the seventh key and discuss patience and fortitude. Emphasize trust as an important element of patience. Remind members that

lifestyle changes happen over time. Encourage them to be patient with themselves and with the process.

11. If time allows, from Day 6 read and discuss any unnecessary keys that may be weighing members down.

12. Close with prayer, including some of the Scripture prayers from Days 6 and 7. Also pray that members will allow Jesus, their Master Key, to unlock the doorways to their successes.

Week Six: Thoughts That Build Success

1. Ask someone in the group who works with computers to explain the concept of programming, or be prepared to explain it yourself. Draw the analogy that our brains are intricate computers that are programmed by the information we put into them. Every computer needs a delete key to erase bad data. We need to add to our programs the correct information from God's Word.

2. Call on two or more members to recite this week's memory verse, Psalm 139:23-24.

3. On the board, write the seven kinds of thoughts that build success as members call out the week's lesson titles. Point out that the battle for our souls is won or lost in our minds. Have volunteers read Romans 8:5; 12:2; 2 Corinthians 4:4; Colossians 3:2.

4. Form three small groups and assign each group one of the following questions: (1) What are some thoughts that hinder success? (2) What are some thoughts that build success? (3) What can I do to develop thoughts/attitudes that build success? Allow five to seven minutes for discussion; then call for reports. Relate the reports to the material in this week's lessons.

5. Based on the small-group reports, lead a discussion of how thoughts can help or hinder a person's progress in the First Place program. Call attention to the activities in Days 2 and 4 that relate to the First Place commitments.

6. Ask for voluntary testimonies from members who feel they have experienced an upsurge in confidence, self-esteem, persistence and/or optimism as a result of the last six weeks of Bible study. Ask: Who feels they have made some wise choices this week? Who has placed their hope in God?

7   Have members privately write down three things that they like about themselves. Without necessarily sharing the things they wrote, have volunteers tell how believing they are special and valued by God influences how they feel about themselves.

8. If you have a wide age span in your group, call on a younger and an older member of the group to tell why they felt now was the right time to be involved in First Place. Ask members if anyone has felt that God has used a child to touch her or his life. Emphasize the importance of being available to God, whatever our physical or spiritual age.

9. Time permitting, discuss the concept of garbage in, garbage out (pp. 91-92). Discuss how/what members are doing to fill their minds with treasure, rather than trash.

10. Read Philippians 4:7-8 and then close with prayer.

Week Seven: Overcoming Leads to Success

1. Call on volunteers to recite this week's memory verse, 1 John 5:4-5. Have members share several ways we use the term "overcome." Conclude that it implies victory: An overcomer is a person who wins out over whatever obstacle is placed in his or her way.

2. Have members turn to Day 1 and ask a volunteer to read the three-point path to victory. Discuss how each of these leads to victory. Discuss: What are some habits members of First Place generally have to overcome? (Thinking of food as a reward, eating too many sugars and fats, failing to exercise, etc.) Emphasize that new habits are built just as older ones: day by day, action by action. Share new habits that you have formed or are forming. Invite others to share their new habits.

3. Ask volunteers to explain the difference between a mistake and a sin.

4. Draw a line down the board to make two columns. Label one "Realistic" and the other "False." Have members call out expectations of the Christian life that fit appropriately in each column. Erase the responses and then ask members to call out expectations in each category— Realistic or False—for the First Place program. Write these in the appropriate columns. Review information about realistic goals in the area of weight loss—one to two pounds per week.

5. Ask members to read their definitions of willfulness from Day 3. Ask if anyone feels rebellious or has felt rebellious about any of the First

Place commitments. Depending on the level of openness and honesty in the group, affirm those who are willing to share that they are struggling with a willful spirit toward God's authority. Spend time in prayer for those who express a need.

6. Lead members to brainstorm limitations (see Day 4, p. 103) that we may feel in reaching First Place goals. Read Acts 4:13. Discuss: How does being with Jesus help us overcome our limitations?

7. Relate Jesus' ability to help us overcome limitations with His ability to help us overcome temptations. Have members share limitations and temptations Jesus faced. Have a volunteer read Hebrews 2:18.

8. Invite members to share the list of doubts expressed in Day 5. Discuss: How do you relate to these doubts? Then ask: How big is a mustard seed? Explain: The *size* of our faith is not as important as the *object* of our faith. With God, all things are possible. **Before the meeting**, if possible bring mustard seeds to class as a visual demonstration. In closing have members sing "Trust and Obey" or a similar hymn or chorus.

9. If time allows, read the reflection statements in Day 7, and then ask members to comment on the questions. Close by using one or more of the Scripture prayers. Pray that members will be overcomers.

Week Eight: Staying on Track to Success

1. Optional: **Before the meeting**, prepare a poster showing traffic-sign shapes without the words. As the meeting begins, have members identify the signs. Use the circle with a slash as an example of how a visual symbol can replace words. Explain: We also depend on sounds to warn us, i.e., sirens and train whistles. Discuss how signs and sounds will keep us on track in our journey through life. Invite volunteers to recite this week's memory verse. Discuss: How do we *hear* God's directions for the way to walk? (Bible study, prayer, worship, Christian friends, etc.) Explain: The more time we spend with the Lord, the more we recognize His ways. Read John 10:14.

2. Discuss: How many stop signs are there between your house and our meeting place? What would happen if you ignored even one of the signs? Review the purpose of spiritual stop signs from Day 1. Remind members that traffic signs are in place for our protection.

3. **Before the meeting**, write the following questions on the board for discussion: (1) What construction project does God want to do in

your life right now? (2) What detours or distractions do you face in cooperating with God's plan? (3) What warning signs have you encountered (i.e., high blood pressure, diabetes, etc.)?

Form groups of three or four. Suggest that they use the material from Days 2 and 3 in their discussion. Remind members of the need for confidentiality in their sharing.

4. Reconvene the whole group. Introduce the material in Day 4 by telling about a traffic ticket or fine that you might have received. Point out what you learned as a result. Discuss: Who are some of the authority figures in our lives who can help us on the pathway to success? How does obeying authority affect our witness to the world? Ask members to evaluate silently whether or not they are good followers. Brainstorm the qualities of a good follower.

5. Ask for synonyms or descriptions of yieldedness. Point out that yieldedness does not make us puppets or robots. God expects us to actively cooperate with Him. Explain: The pathway to success requires walking. It is not an escalator or conveyor belt! Mention the examples of yieldedness in Day 5 that involve proactive choices. Read the comments (p. 122) in Day 6 on being yielded to our heavenly Father.

6. If time allows, read the statements about crossroads in Day 7 and ask members to share about any that they face. As members bow for prayer, offer encouragement to those who feel they have gotten off track. Remind them that God's mercies are new every morning (see Lamentations 3:22-23). Close with prayer.

Week Nine: Managing Success

1. Find a current-event story about a successful person who is not managing success well. Or use the following case study:

The executive officer of a local corporation who committed suicide yesterday buckled under the stress of day-to-day corporate business, according to his son. The son expressed shock that his father ended his life. "It wasn't my father's personality to do something like this," he added.

Discuss: What factors might lead someone to manage success so poorly that he would commit suicide at the height of his successful career?

2. Ask members to share about someone that they know who has managed success well and to mention the factors that seemed to contribute to his or her ongoing success. Write these factors on the board. Have members recall the ways to manage success that are suggested by this week's lesson titles. Add these to the list.

3. Ask a volunteer to recite this week's memory verse. Emphasize the role of the Holy Spirit in guarding our hearts. Discuss: What is the good deposit Paul was referencing in 2 Timothy 1:14? (Sound doctrine.) What good deposits do you have thus far in First Place? (Weight loss, physical fitness, Scripture memory, etc.)

4. Form two groups. Assign one group the qualities of pride, self-righteousness and envy. Assign the other group the qualities of healthy self-esteem, humility and generosity. Ask groups to share from Days 1 and 2 how these qualities help or hinder managing success. After three to five minutes, call for reports.

5. **Before the meeting**, procure a working flashlight. Demonstrate the effect of a flashlight with and without batteries. Ask a volunteer to draw a parallel to our success in the Christian life and First Place. Read the concluding thoughts from Day 3 (p. 131).

6. Allow ample time for members to share the testimonies that they wrote on Day 4. If you have a large group, form smaller groups of three to five in which to share the testimonies. Affirm members by pointing out that small steps toward long-range goals are as worthwhile as dramatic accomplishments.

7. Reference the challenge in Day 5 to seek new directions. Explain: Moving on to new goals demonstrates our commitment to continue to follow God wherever He leads. If we give up or quit at a certain point, we have chosen to follow only a portion of the pathway to success.

8. Time permitting, refer to the outline for managing success as shared in Day 7. Select members to read each point and the Scripture prayer with it. Let members know they can participate, even if they did not read it.

9. Lead the group in a time of thanksgiving and praise to God. Call on volunteers to read Jude 24-25 and Revelation 4:11 from Day 4. Have the group offer sentence prayers of praise and thanksgiving.

Week Ten: Called to Success

1. **Before the meeting,** make this final session a festive celebration of the royal priesthood of Christ's followers by decorating with purple for royalty and with crowns for everyone. Adapt the closing activities to meet the needs of your group.

2. Call on volunteers to recite this week's Scripture memory verse. Have members define or give synonyms for the keywords from the verse: "chosen," "royal," "holy," "belonging" and "called." Discuss: What is our purpose in being called to success? (To praise God.) What are we called from and to? (From darkness to light.)

3. Call attention to the royal decorations. Ask members to describe what life as a child of a king would be like. Apply these descriptions to our lives as children of the heavenly King. Explain: Today we will see how Jesus is our perfect example of a child of the King. Discuss: What did He do that demonstrates how a child of the King lives? Have members turn to Day 1 and review the relationship between choosing God's way and blessings versus choosing unhealthy lifestyle choices and death. Ask a volunteer to read the choice Jesus made in Matthew 26:39. Discuss: How did Jesus' choice result in blessing? After several responses, read Ephesians 1:3. Lead the group to summarize the lifestyle choices of a child of the King.

4. Review the process for becoming a new creation in Christ from Day 2. Read Philippians 2:5-8. Compare Jesus' willingness to humble Himself with our need to admit limitations and allow God to control.

5. Review Day 3. Ask members to give examples of how Jesus stood firm in the face of adverse circumstances. Mention His reliance on Scripture and prayer. Read John 6:38. Discuss: What motivated Jesus to stand firm? Should we have the same motivation in our lifestyle choices?

6. Invite volunteers to share what they wrote in Day 3 to describe children of light and children of darkness. Have someone read Colossians 1:12-14 and summarize how we become citizens of the Kingdom of light. Emphasize living in such a way that Christ's light shines through us into a world of darkness.

7. Review Day 4. Have someone read John 19:30. Relate Jesus' words to crossing the finish line in Day 5. Conclude by reading 1 Corinthians 15:56-57 to praise Jesus' victory over sin and death. Lead the group to summarize how Jesus demonstrates how a child of the King lives.

8. If time allows, review the list of weekly titles in Day 6. Invite members to recite the memory verses for each week in unison.

9. Discuss the pathway to success as mentioned in Day 7. Read the quote by Roy Lessin (p. 159). Thank the group for their faithfulness and encourage members to continue the journey on the high road, the true pathway to success.

10. Join hands, close with sentence prayers, and read the Ephesians 3:14-21 Scripture prayer from Day 7.

PERSONAL WEIGHT RECORD

Week	Weight	+ or -	Goal This Session	Pounds to Goal
1				
2				
3				
4				
5				
6				
7				
8				
9				
10				
11				
12				
13				
Final				

Beginning Measurements

Waist_____ Hips_____ Thighs_____ Chest_____

Ending Measurements

Waist_____ Hips_____ Thighs_____ Chest_____

COMMITMENT RECORDS

How to Fill Out a Commitment Record

The Commitment Record (CR) is an aid for you in keeping track of your accomplishments. Begin a new CR on the morning of the day your class meets. This ensures that your CR is complete before your next meeting. Turn in the CR weekly to your leader.

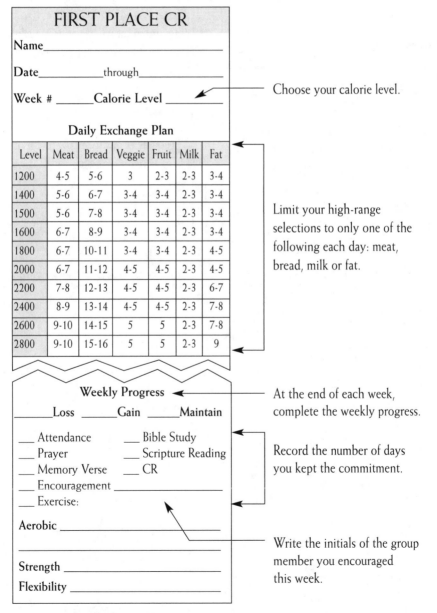

FIRST PLACE CR

Name_____

Date_____through_____

Week # _____Calorie Level _____

Choose your calorie level.

Daily Exchange Plan

Level	Meat	Bread	Veggie	Fruit	Milk	Fat
1200	4-5	5-6	3	2-3	2-3	3-4
1400	5-6	6-7	3-4	3-4	2-3	3-4
1500	5-6	7-8	3-4	3-4	2-3	3-4
1600	6-7	8-9	3-4	3-4	2-3	3-4
1800	6-7	10-11	3-4	3-4	2-3	4-5
2000	6-7	11-12	4-5	4-5	2-3	4-5
2200	7-8	12-13	4-5	4-5	2-3	6-7
2400	8-9	13-14	4-5	4-5	2-3	7-8
2600	9-10	14-15	5	5	2-3	7-8
2800	9-10	15-16	5	5	2-3	9

Limit your high-range selections to only one of the following each day: meat, bread, milk or fat.

Weekly Progress

_____Loss _____Gain _____Maintain

___ Attendance   ___ Bible Study
___ Prayer   ___ Scripture Reading
___ Memory Verse   ___ CR
___ Encouragement _____
___ Exercise:

Aerobic _____

_____

Strength _____

Flexibility _____

At the end of each week, complete the weekly progress.

Record the number of days you kept the commitment.

Write the initials of the group member you encouraged this week.

DAY 7: Date _____

Morning _____
_____
_____
Midday _____
_____
_____
Evening _____
_____
_____
Snacks _____
_____
_____

___ Meat _____ ☐ Prayer
___ Bread _____ ☐ Bible Study
___ Vegetable ____ ☐ Scripture Reading
___ Fruit _____ ☐ Memory Verse
___ Milk _____ ☐ Encouragement
___ Fat _____ ☐ Water_____
Exercise:
Aerobic _____
_____
Strength _____
Flexibility _____

List the foods you have eaten. On this condensed CR it is not necessary to exchange each food choice. It will be the responsibility of each member that the tally marks you list below are accurate regarding each food choice. If you are unsure of an exchange, check the Live-It section of your copy of the *Member's Guide*.

List the daily food exchange choices to the left of the food groups.

Use tally marks for the actual food and water consumed.

Check off commitments completed. Use tally marks to record each 8-oz. serving of water.

List type and duration of exercise.

Name _____

Date _____ through _____

Week # _____ Calorie Level _____

Daily Exchange Plan

Level	Meat	Bread	Veggie	Fruit	Milk	Fat
1200	4-5	5-6	3	2-3	2-3	3-4
1400	5-6	6-7	3-4	3-4	2-3	3-4
1500	5-6	7-8	3-4	3-4	2-3	3-4
1600	6-7	8-9	3-4	3-4	2-3	3-4
1800	6-7	10-11	3-4	3-4	2-3	4-5
2000	6-7	11-12	4-5	4-5	2-3	4-5
2200	7-8	12-13	4-5	4-5	2-3	6-7
2400	8-9	13-14	4-5	4-5	2-3	7-8
2600	9-10	14-15	5	5	2-3	7-8
2800	9-10	15-16	5	5	2-3	9

You may always choose the high range of vegetables and fruits. Limit your high range selections to only one of the following: meat, bread, milk or fat.

Weekly Progress

_____ Loss _____ Gain _____ Maintain

_____ Attendance _____ Bible Study
_____ Prayer _____ Scripture Reading
_____ Memory Verse _____ CR
_____ Encouragement:
_____ Exercise
Aerobic _____

Strength _____
Flexibility _____

DAY 7: Date _____

Morning _____
_____

Midday _____
_____

Evening _____
_____

Snacks _____
_____

_____ Meat   ☐ Prayer
_____ Bread   ☐ Bible Study
_____ Vegetable   ☐ Scripture Reading
_____ Fruit   ☐ Memory Verse
_____ Milk   ☐ Encouragement
_____ Fat   _____ Water

Exercise
Aerobic _____

Strength _____
Flexibility _____

DAY 6: Date _____

Morning _____
_____

Midday _____
_____

Evening _____
_____

Snacks _____
_____

_____ Meat   ☐ Prayer
_____ Bread   ☐ Bible Study
_____ Vegetable   ☐ Scripture Reading
_____ Fruit   ☐ Memory Verse
_____ Milk   ☐ Encouragement
_____ Fat   _____ Water

Exercise
Aerobic _____

Strength _____
Flexibility _____

DAY 5: Date _____

Morning _____
_____

Midday _____
_____

Evening _____
_____

Snacks _____
_____

_____ Meat   ☐ Prayer
_____ Bread   ☐ Bible Study
_____ Vegetable   ☐ Scripture Reading
_____ Fruit   ☐ Memory Verse
_____ Milk   ☐ Encouragement
_____ Fat   _____ Water

Exercise
Aerobic _____

Strength _____
Flexibility _____

DAY 1: Date _____

Morning _____

Midday _____

Evening _____

Snacks _____

Meat _____	☐ Prayer
Bread _____	☐ Bible Study
Vegetable _____	☐ Scripture Reading
Fruit _____	☐ Memory Verse
Milk _____	☐ Encouragement
Fat _____ Water _____	

Exercise
Aerobic _____

Strength _____

Flexibility _____

DAY 2: Date _____

Morning _____

Midday _____

Evening _____

Snacks _____

Meat _____	☐ Prayer
Bread _____	☐ Bible Study
Vegetable _____	☐ Scripture Reading
Fruit _____	☐ Memory Verse
Milk _____	☐ Encouragement
Fat _____ Water _____	

Exercise
Aerobic _____

Strength _____

Flexibility _____

DAY 3: Date _____

Morning _____

Midday _____

Evening _____

Snacks _____

Meat _____	☐ Prayer
Bread _____	☐ Bible Study
Vegetable _____	☐ Scripture Reading
Fruit _____	☐ Memory Verse
Milk _____	☐ Encouragement
Fat _____ Water _____	

Exercise
Aerobic _____

Strength _____

Flexibility _____

DAY 4: Date _____

Morning _____

Midday _____

Evening _____

Snacks _____

Meat _____	☐ Prayer
Bread _____	☐ Bible Study
Vegetable _____	☐ Scripture Reading
Fruit _____	☐ Memory Verse
Milk _____	☐ Encouragement
Fat _____ Water _____	

Exercise
Aerobic _____

Strength _____

Flexibility _____

Name _____

Date _____ through _____

Week # _____ Calorie Level _____

Daily Exchange Plan

Level	Meat	Bread	Veggie	Fruit	Milk	Fat
1200	4-5	5-6	3	2-3	2-3	3-4
1400	5-6	6-7	3-4	3-4	2-3	3-4
1500	5-6	7-8	3-4	3-4	2-3	3-4
1600	6-7	8-9	3-4	3-4	2-3	3-4
1800	6-7	10-11	3-4	3-4	2-3	4-5
2000	6-7	11-12	4-5	4-5	2-3	4-5
2200	7-8	12-13	4-5	4-5	2-3	6-7
2400	8-9	13-14	4-5	4-5	2-3	7-8
2600	9-10	14-15	5	5	2-3	7-8
2800	9-10	15-16	5	5	2-3	9

You may always choose the high range of vegetables and fruits. Limit your high range selections to only one of the following: meat, bread, milk or fat.

Weekly Progress

_____ Loss _____ Gain _____ Maintain

_____ Attendance _____ Bible Study
_____ Prayer _____ Scripture Reading
_____ Memory Verse _____ CR
_____ Encouragement:
_____ Exercise
Aerobic

Strength _____
Flexibility _____

DAY 5: Date _____

Morning _____

Midday _____

Evening _____

Snacks _____

_____ Meat _____
_____ Bread _____
_____ Vegetable _____
_____ Fruit _____
_____ Milk _____
_____ Fat _____ Water _____

☐ Prayer
☐ Bible Study
☐ Scripture Reading
☐ Memory Verse
☐ Encouragement

Exercise
Aerobic _____

Strength _____
Flexibility _____

DAY 6: Date _____

Morning _____

Midday _____

Evening _____

Snacks _____

_____ Meat _____
_____ Bread _____
_____ Vegetable _____
_____ Fruit _____
_____ Milk _____
_____ Fat _____ Water _____

☐ Prayer
☐ Bible Study
☐ Scripture Reading
☐ Memory Verse
☐ Encouragement

Exercise
Aerobic _____

Strength _____
Flexibility _____

DAY 7: Date _____

Morning _____

Midday _____

Evening _____

Snacks _____

_____ Meat _____
_____ Bread _____
_____ Vegetable _____
_____ Fruit _____
_____ Milk _____
_____ Fat _____ Water _____

☐ Prayer
☐ Bible Study
☐ Scripture Reading
☐ Memory Verse
☐ Encouragement

Exercise
Aerobic _____

Strength _____
Flexibility _____

DAY 1: Date _____

Morning _____

Midday _____

Evening _____

Snacks _____

___ Meat	☐ Prayer
___ Bread	☐ Bible Study
___ Vegetable	☐ Scripture Reading
___ Fruit	☐ Memory Verse
___ Milk	☐ Encouragement
___ Fat	___ Water

Exercise
Aerobic _____
Strength _____
Flexibility _____

DAY 2: Date _____

Morning _____

Midday _____

Evening _____

Snacks _____

___ Meat	☐ Prayer
___ Bread	☐ Bible Study
___ Vegetable	☐ Scripture Reading
___ Fruit	☐ Memory Verse
___ Milk	☐ Encouragement
___ Fat	___ Water

Exercise
Aerobic _____
Strength _____
Flexibility _____

DAY 3: Date _____

Morning _____

Midday _____

Evening _____

Snacks _____

___ Meat	☐ Prayer
___ Bread	☐ Bible Study
___ Vegetable	☐ Scripture Reading
___ Fruit	☐ Memory Verse
___ Milk	☐ Encouragement
___ Fat	___ Water

Exercise
Aerobic _____
Strength _____
Flexibility _____

DAY 4: Date _____

Morning _____

Midday _____

Evening _____

Snacks _____

___ Meat	☐ Prayer
___ Bread	☐ Bible Study
___ Vegetable	☐ Scripture Reading
___ Fruit	☐ Memory Verse
___ Milk	☐ Encouragement
___ Fat	___ Water

Exercise
Aerobic _____
Strength _____
Flexibility _____

FIRST PLACE CR

Name _____

Date _____ through _____

Week # _____ Calorie Level _____

Daily Exchange Plan

Level	Meat	Bread	Veggie	Fruit	Milk	Fat
1200	4-5	5-6	3	2-3	2-3	3-4
1400	5-6	6-7	3-4	3-4	2-3	3-4
1500	5-6	7-8	3-4	3-4	2-3	3-4
1600	6-7	8-9	3-4	3-4	2-3	3-4
1800	6-7	10-11	3-4	3-4	2-3	4-5
2000	6-7	11-12	4-5	4-5	2-3	4-5
2200	7-8	12-13	4-5	4-5	2-3	6-7
2400	8-9	13-14	4-5	4-5	2-3	7-8
2600	9-10	14-15	5	5	2-3	7-8
2800	9-10	15-16	5	5	2-3	9

You may always choose the high range of vegetables and fruits. Limit your high range selections to only one of the following: meat, bread, milk or fat.

Weekly Progress

_____ Loss _____ Gain _____ Maintain

_____ Attendance _____ Bible Study
_____ Prayer _____ Scripture Reading
_____ Memory Verse _____ CR
_____ Encouragement:
_____ Exercise
Aerobic _____

Strength _____
Flexibility _____

DAY 5: Date _____

Morning _____

Midday _____

Evening _____

Snacks _____

_____ Meat   ☐ Prayer
_____ Bread   ☐ Bible Study
_____ Vegetable   ☐ Scripture Reading
_____ Fruit   ☐ Memory Verse
_____ Milk   ☐ Encouragement
_____ Fat   ☐ Water

Exercise
Aerobic _____

Strength _____
Flexibility _____

DAY 6: Date _____

Morning _____

Midday _____

Evening _____

Snacks _____

_____ Meat   ☐ Prayer
_____ Bread   ☐ Bible Study
_____ Vegetable   ☐ Scripture Reading
_____ Fruit   ☐ Memory Verse
_____ Milk   ☐ Encouragement
_____ Fat   ☐ Water

Exercise
Aerobic _____

Strength _____
Flexibility _____

DAY 7: Date _____

Morning _____

Midday _____

Evening _____

Snacks _____

_____ Meat   ☐ Prayer
_____ Bread   ☐ Bible Study
_____ Vegetable   ☐ Scripture Reading
_____ Fruit   ☐ Memory Verse
_____ Milk   ☐ Encouragement
_____ Fat   ☐ Water

Exercise
Aerobic _____

Strength _____
Flexibility _____

DAY 1: Date _____

Morning _____

Midday _____

Evening _____

Snacks _____

____ Meat	☐ Prayer
____ Bread	☐ Bible Study
____ Vegetable	☐ Scripture Reading
____ Fruit	☐ Memory Verse
____ Milk	☐ Encouragement
____ Fat	____ Water

Exercise
Aerobic _____
Strength _____
Flexibility _____

DAY 2: Date _____

Morning _____

Midday _____

Evening _____

Snacks _____

____ Meat	☐ Prayer
____ Bread	☐ Bible Study
____ Vegetable	☐ Scripture Reading
____ Fruit	☐ Memory Verse
____ Milk	☐ Encouragement
____ Fat	____ Water

Exercise
Aerobic _____
Strength _____
Flexibility _____

DAY 3: Date _____

Morning _____

Midday _____

Evening _____

Snacks _____

____ Meat	☐ Prayer
____ Bread	☐ Bible Study
____ Vegetable	☐ Scripture Reading
____ Fruit	☐ Memory Verse
____ Milk	☐ Encouragement
____ Fat	____ Water

Exercise
Aerobic _____
Strength _____
Flexibility _____

DAY 4: Date _____

Morning _____

Midday _____

Evening _____

Snacks _____

____ Meat	☐ Prayer
____ Bread	☐ Bible Study
____ Vegetable	☐ Scripture Reading
____ Fruit	☐ Memory Verse
____ Milk	☐ Encouragement
____ Fat	____ Water

Exercise
Aerobic _____
Strength _____
Flexibility _____

FIRST PLACE CR

Name _____

Date _____ through _____

Week # _____ Calorie Level _____

Daily Exchange Plan

Level	Meat	Bread	Veggie	Fruit	Milk	Fat
1200	4-5	5-6	3	2-3	2-3	3-4
1400	5-6	6-7	3-4	3-4	2-3	3-4
1500	5-6	7-8	3-4	3-4	2-3	3-4
1600	6-7	8-9	3-4	3-4	2-3	3-4
1800	6-7	10-11	3-4	3-4	2-3	4-5
2000	6-7	11-12	4-5	4-5	2-3	4-5
2200	7-8	12-13	4-5	4-5	2-3	6-7
2400	8-9	13-14	4-5	4-5	2-3	7-8
2600	9-10	14-15	5	5	2-3	7-8
2800	9-10	15-16	5	5	2-3	9

You may always choose the high range of vegetables and fruits. Limit your high range selections to only one of the following: meat, bread, milk or fat.

Weekly Progress

_____ Loss _____ Gain _____ Maintain

_____ Attendance _____ Bible Study
_____ Prayer _____ Scripture Reading
_____ Memory Verse _____ CR
_____ Encouragement:
_____ Exercise
Aerobic _____

Strength _____
Flexibility _____

DAY 5: Date _____

Morning _____

Midday _____

Evening _____

Snacks _____

_____ Meat   ☐ Prayer
_____ Bread   ☐ Bible Study
_____ Vegetable   ☐ Scripture Reading
_____ Fruit   ☐ Memory Verse
_____ Milk   ☐ Encouragement
_____ Fat   _____ Water

Exercise
Aerobic _____

Strength _____
Flexibility _____

DAY 6: Date _____

Morning _____

Midday _____

Evening _____

Snacks _____

_____ Meat   ☐ Prayer
_____ Bread   ☐ Bible Study
_____ Vegetable   ☐ Scripture Reading
_____ Fruit   ☐ Memory Verse
_____ Milk   ☐ Encouragement
_____ Fat   _____ Water

Exercise
Aerobic _____

Strength _____
Flexibility _____

DAY 7: Date _____

Morning _____

Midday _____

Evening _____

Snacks _____

_____ Meat   ☐ Prayer
_____ Bread   ☐ Bible Study
_____ Vegetable   ☐ Scripture Reading
_____ Fruit   ☐ Memory Verse
_____ Milk   ☐ Encouragement
_____ Fat   _____ Water

Exercise
Aerobic _____

Strength _____
Flexibility _____

DAY 1: Date _____

Morning _____

Midday _____

Evening _____

Snacks _____

☐ Prayer ____ Meat _____
☐ Bible Study ____ Bread _____
☐ Scripture Reading ____ Vegetable _____
☐ Memory Verse ____ Fruit _____
☐ Encouragement ____ Milk _____
____ Fat _____
____ Water _____

Exercise
Aerobic _____
Strength _____
Flexibility _____

DAY 2: Date _____

Morning _____

Midday _____

Evening _____

Snacks _____

☐ Prayer ____ Meat _____
☐ Bible Study ____ Bread _____
☐ Scripture Reading ____ Vegetable _____
☐ Memory Verse ____ Fruit _____
☐ Encouragement ____ Milk _____
____ Fat _____
____ Water _____

Exercise
Aerobic _____
Strength _____
Flexibility _____

DAY 3: Date _____

Morning _____

Midday _____

Evening _____

Snacks _____

☐ Prayer ____ Meat _____
☐ Bible Study ____ Bread _____
☐ Scripture Reading ____ Vegetable _____
☐ Memory Verse ____ Fruit _____
☐ Encouragement ____ Milk _____
____ Fat _____
____ Water _____

Exercise
Aerobic _____
Strength _____
Flexibility _____

DAY 4: Date _____

Morning _____

Midday _____

Evening _____

Snacks _____

☐ Prayer ____ Meat _____
☐ Bible Study ____ Bread _____
☐ Scripture Reading ____ Vegetable _____
☐ Memory Verse ____ Fruit _____
☐ Encouragement ____ Milk _____
____ Fat _____
____ Water _____

Exercise
Aerobic _____
Strength _____
Flexibility _____

FIRST PLACE CR

Name _____

Date _____ through _____

Week # _____ Calorie Level _____

Daily Exchange Plan

Level	Meat	Bread	Veggie	Fruit	Milk	Fat
1200	4-5	5-6	3	2-3	2-3	3-4
1400	5-6	6-7	3-4	3-4	2-3	3-4
1500	5-6	7-8	3-4	3-4	2-3	3-4
1600	6-7	8-9	3-4	3-4	2-3	3-4
1800	6-7	10-11	3-4	3-4	2-3	4-5
2000	6-7	11-12	4-5	4-5	2-3	4-5
2200	7-8	12-13	4-5	4-5	2-3	6-7
2400	8-9	13-14	4-5	4-5	2-3	7-8
2600	9-10	14-15	5	5	2-3	7-8
2800	9-10	15-16	5	5	2-3	9

You may always choose the high range of vegetables and fruits. Limit your high range selections to only one of the following: meat, bread, milk or fat.

Weekly Progress

_____ Loss _____ Gain _____ Maintain

_____ Attendance _____ Bible Study

_____ Prayer _____ Scripture Reading

_____ Memory Verse _____ CR

_____ Encouragement:

_____ Exercise

_____ Aerobic

_____ Strength

_____ Flexibility

DAY 7: Date _____

Morning _____

Midday _____

Evening _____

Snacks _____

_____ Meat □ Prayer
_____ Bread □ Bible Study
_____ Vegetable □ Scripture Reading
_____ Fruit □ Memory Verse
_____ Milk □ Encouragement
_____ Fat _____ Water

Exercise
Aerobic _____

Strength _____
Flexibility _____

DAY 6: Date _____

Morning _____

Midday _____

Evening _____

Snacks _____

_____ Meat □ Prayer
_____ Bread □ Bible Study
_____ Vegetable □ Scripture Reading
_____ Fruit □ Memory Verse
_____ Milk □ Encouragement
_____ Fat _____ Water

Exercise
Aerobic _____

Strength _____
Flexibility _____

DAY 5: Date _____

Morning _____

Midday _____

Evening _____

Snacks _____

_____ Meat □ Prayer
_____ Bread □ Bible Study
_____ Vegetable □ Scripture Reading
_____ Fruit □ Memory Verse
_____ Milk □ Encouragement
_____ Fat _____ Water

Exercise
Aerobic _____

Strength _____
Flexibility _____

DAY 1: Date _____

Morning _____

Midday _____

Evening _____

Snacks _____

____ Meat ____   ☐ Prayer
____ Bread ____   ☐ Bible Study
____ Vegetable ____ ☐ Scripture Reading
____ Fruit ____   ☐ Memory Verse
____ Milk ____   ☐ Encouragement
____ Fat ____ Water ____

Exercise
Aerobic _____
Strength _____
Flexibility _____

DAY 2: Date _____

Morning _____

Midday _____

Evening _____

Snacks _____

____ Meat ____   ☐ Prayer
____ Bread ____   ☐ Bible Study
____ Vegetable ____ ☐ Scripture Reading
____ Fruit ____   ☐ Memory Verse
____ Milk ____   ☐ Encouragement
____ Fat ____ Water ____

Exercise
Aerobic _____
Strength _____
Flexibility _____

DAY 3: Date _____

Morning _____

Midday _____

Evening _____

Snacks _____

____ Meat ____   ☐ Prayer
____ Bread ____   ☐ Bible Study
____ Vegetable ____ ☐ Scripture Reading
____ Fruit ____   ☐ Memory Verse
____ Milk ____   ☐ Encouragement
____ Fat ____ Water ____

Exercise
Aerobic _____
Strength _____
Flexibility _____

DAY 4: Date _____

Morning _____

Midday _____

Evening _____

Snacks _____

____ Meat ____   ☐ Prayer
____ Bread ____   ☐ Bible Study
____ Vegetable ____ ☐ Scripture Reading
____ Fruit ____   ☐ Memory Verse
____ Milk ____   ☐ Encouragement
____ Fat ____ Water ____

Exercise
Aerobic _____
Strength _____
Flexibility _____

FIRST PLACE CR

Name _____

Date _____ through _____

Week # _____ Calorie Level _____

Daily Exchange Plan

Level	Meat	Bread	Veggie	Fruit	Milk	Fat
1200	4-5	5-6	3	2-3	2-3	3-4
1400	5-6	6-7	3-4	3-4	2-3	3-4
1500	5-6	7-8	3-4	3-4	2-3	3-4
1600	6-7	8-9	3-4	3-4	2-3	3-4
1800	6-7	10-11	3-4	3-4	2-3	4-5
2000	6-7	11-12	4-5	4-5	2-3	4-5
2200	7-8	12-13	4-5	4-5	2-3	6-7
2400	8-9	13-14	4-5	4-5	2-3	7-8
2600	9-10	14-15	5	5	2-3	7-8
2800	9-10	15-16	5	5	2-3	9

You may always choose the high range of vegetables and fruits. Limit your high range selections to only one of the following: meat, bread, milk or fat.

Weekly Progress

_____ Loss _____ Gain _____ Maintain

_____ Attendance _____ Bible Study

_____ Prayer _____ Scripture Reading

_____ Memory Verse _____ CR

_____ Encouragement:

_____ Exercise

_____ Aerobic

_____ Strength

_____ Flexibility

DAY 7: Date _____

Morning _____

Midday _____

Evening _____

Snacks _____

_____ Meat □ Prayer
_____ Bread □ Bible Study
_____ Vegetable □ Scripture Reading
_____ Fruit □ Memory Verse
_____ Milk □ Encouragement
_____ Fat Water _____

Exercise
Aerobic _____

Strength _____
Flexibility _____

DAY 6: Date _____

Morning _____

Midday _____

Evening _____

Snacks _____

_____ Meat □ Prayer
_____ Bread □ Bible Study
_____ Vegetable □ Scripture Reading
_____ Fruit □ Memory Verse
_____ Milk □ Encouragement
_____ Fat Water _____

Exercise
Aerobic _____

Strength _____
Flexibility _____

DAY 5: Date _____

Morning _____

Midday _____

Evening _____

Snacks _____

_____ Meat □ Prayer
_____ Bread □ Bible Study
_____ Vegetable □ Scripture Reading
_____ Fruit □ Memory Verse
_____ Milk □ Encouragement
_____ Fat Water _____

Exercise
Aerobic _____

Strength _____
Flexibility _____

DAY 1: Date _____   DAY 2: Date _____   DAY 3: Date _____   DAY 4: Date _____

DAY 1

Morning _____

Midday _____

Evening _____

Snacks _____

___ Meat _____   ☐ Prayer
___ Bread _____   ☐ Bible Study
___ Vegetable _____   ☐ Scripture Reading
___ Fruit _____   ☐ Memory Verse
___ Milk _____   ☐ Encouragement
___ Fat _____   ___ Water _____

Exercise
Aerobic _____
Strength _____
Flexibility _____

DAY 2

Morning _____

Midday _____

Evening _____

Snacks _____

___ Meat _____   ☐ Prayer
___ Bread _____   ☐ Bible Study
___ Vegetable _____   ☐ Scripture Reading
___ Fruit _____   ☐ Memory Verse
___ Milk _____   ☐ Encouragement
___ Fat _____   ___ Water _____

Exercise
Aerobic _____
Strength _____
Flexibility _____

DAY 3

Morning _____

Midday _____

Evening _____

Snacks _____

___ Meat _____   ☐ Prayer
___ Bread _____   ☐ Bible Study
___ Vegetable _____   ☐ Scripture Reading
___ Fruit _____   ☐ Memory Verse
___ Milk _____   ☐ Encouragement
___ Fat _____   ___ Water _____

Exercise
Aerobic _____
Strength _____
Flexibility _____

DAY 4

Morning _____

Midday _____

Evening _____

Snacks _____

___ Meat _____   ☐ Prayer
___ Bread _____   ☐ Bible Study
___ Vegetable _____   ☐ Scripture Reading
___ Fruit _____   ☐ Memory Verse
___ Milk _____   ☐ Encouragement
___ Fat _____   ___ Water _____

Exercise
Aerobic _____
Strength _____
Flexibility _____

FIRST PLACE CR

Name _____

Date _____ through _____

Week # _____ Calorie Level _____

Daily Exchange Plan

Level	Meat	Bread	Veggie	Fruit	Milk	Fat
1200	4-5	5-6	3	2-3	2-3	3-4
1400	5-6	6-7	3-4	3-4	2-3	3-4
1500	5-6	7-8	3-4	3-4	2-3	3-4
1600	6-7	8-9	3-4	3-4	2-3	3-4
1800	6-7	10-11	3-4	3-4	2-3	4-5
2000	6-7	11-12	4-5	4-5	2-3	4-5
2200	7-8	12-13	4-5	4-5	2-3	6-7
2400	8-9	13-14	4-5	4-5	2-3	7-8
2600	9-10	14-15	5	5	2-3	7-8
2800	9-10	15-16	5	5	2-3	9

You may always choose the high range of vegetables and fruits. Limit your high range selections to only one of the following: meat, bread, milk or fat.

Weekly Progress

_____ Loss   _____ Gain   _____ Maintain

_____ Attendance   _____ Bible Study
_____ Prayer   _____ Scripture Reading
_____ Memory Verse   _____ CR
_____ Encouragement:
_____ Exercise
_____ Aerobic
_____ Strength
_____ Flexibility

DAY 5: Date _____

Morning _____

Midday _____

Evening _____

Snacks _____

_____ Meat   ☐ Prayer
_____ Bread   ☐ Bible Study
_____ Vegetable   ☐ Scripture Reading
_____ Fruit   ☐ Memory Verse
_____ Milk   ☐ Encouragement
_____ Fat   _____ Water

Exercise
Aerobic _____

Strength _____
Flexibility _____

DAY 6: Date _____

Morning _____

Midday _____

Evening _____

Snacks _____

_____ Meat   ☐ Prayer
_____ Bread   ☐ Bible Study
_____ Vegetable   ☐ Scripture Reading
_____ Fruit   ☐ Memory Verse
_____ Milk   ☐ Encouragement
_____ Fat   _____ Water

Exercise
Aerobic _____

Strength _____
Flexibility _____

DAY 7: Date _____

Morning _____

Midday _____

Evening _____

Snacks _____

_____ Meat   ☐ Prayer
_____ Bread   ☐ Bible Study
_____ Vegetable   ☐ Scripture Reading
_____ Fruit   ☐ Memory Verse
_____ Milk   ☐ Encouragement
_____ Fat   _____ Water

Exercise
Aerobic _____

Strength _____
Flexibility _____

DAY 1: Date _____

Morning _____

Midday _____

Evening _____

Snacks _____

____ Meat	☐ Prayer
____ Bread	☐ Bible Study
____ Vegetable	☐ Scripture Reading
____ Fruit	☐ Memory Verse
____ Milk	☐ Encouragement
____ Fat	____ Water

Exercise
Aerobic _____
Strength _____
Flexibility _____

DAY 2: Date _____

Morning _____

Midday _____

Evening _____

Snacks _____

____ Meat	☐ Prayer
____ Bread	☐ Bible Study
____ Vegetable	☐ Scripture Reading
____ Fruit	☐ Memory Verse
____ Milk	☐ Encouragement
____ Fat	____ Water

Exercise
Aerobic _____
Strength _____
Flexibility _____

DAY 3: Date _____

Morning _____

Midday _____

Evening _____

Snacks _____

____ Meat	☐ Prayer
____ Bread	☐ Bible Study
____ Vegetable	☐ Scripture Reading
____ Fruit	☐ Memory Verse
____ Milk	☐ Encouragement
____ Fat	____ Water

Exercise
Aerobic _____
Strength _____
Flexibility _____

DAY 4: Date _____

Morning _____

Midday _____

Evening _____

Snacks _____

____ Meat	☐ Prayer
____ Bread	☐ Bible Study
____ Vegetable	☐ Scripture Reading
____ Fruit	☐ Memory Verse
____ Milk	☐ Encouragement
____ Fat	____ Water

Exercise
Aerobic _____
Strength _____
Flexibility _____

FIRST PLACE CR

Name _____

Date _____ through _____

Week # _____ Calorie Level _____

Daily Exchange Plan

Level	Meat	Bread	Veggie	Fruit	Milk	Fat
1200	4-5	5-6	3	2-3	2-3	3-4
1400	5-6	6-7	3-4	3-4	2-3	3-4
1500	5-6	7-8	3-4	3-4	2-3	3-4
1600	6-7	8-9	3-4	3-4	2-3	3-4
1800	6-7	10-11	3-4	3-4	2-3	4-5
2000	6-7	11-12	4-5	4-5	2-3	4-5
2200	7-8	12-13	4-5	4-5	2-3	6-7
2400	8-9	13-14	4-5	4-5	2-3	7-8
2600	9-10	14-15	5	5	2-3	7-8
2800	9-10	15-16	5	5	2-3	9

You may always choose the high range of vegetables and fruits. Limit your high range selections to only one of the following: meat, bread, milk or fat.

Weekly Progress

_____ Loss _____ Gain _____ Maintain

_____ Attendance _____ Bible Study
_____ Prayer _____ Scripture Reading
_____ Memory Verse _____ CR

Encouragement: _____

Exercise
Aerobic _____

Strength _____
Flexibility _____

DAY 7: Date _____

Morning _____

Midday _____

Evening _____

Snacks _____

_____ Meat ☐ Prayer
_____ Bread ☐ Bible Study
_____ Vegetable ☐ Scripture Reading
_____ Fruit ☐ Memory Verse
_____ Milk ☐ Encouragement
_____ Fat Water _____

Exercise
Aerobic _____

Strength _____
Flexibility _____

DAY 6: Date _____

Morning _____

Midday _____

Evening _____

Snacks _____

_____ Meat ☐ Prayer
_____ Bread ☐ Bible Study
_____ Vegetable ☐ Scripture Reading
_____ Fruit ☐ Memory Verse
_____ Milk ☐ Encouragement
_____ Fat Water _____

Exercise
Aerobic _____

Strength _____
Flexibility _____

DAY 5: Date _____

Morning _____

Midday _____

Evening _____

Snacks _____

_____ Meat ☐ Prayer
_____ Bread ☐ Bible Study
_____ Vegetable ☐ Scripture Reading
_____ Fruit ☐ Memory Verse
_____ Milk ☐ Encouragement
_____ Fat Water _____

Exercise
Aerobic _____

Strength _____
Flexibility _____

DAY 1:

Morning _____

Midday _____

Evening _____

Snacks _____

____ Meat	☐ Prayer
____ Bread	☐ Bible Study
____ Vegetable	☐ Scripture Reading
____ Fruit	☐ Memory Verse
____ Milk	☐ Encouragement
____ Fat	____ Water

Exercise
Aerobic _____
Strength _____
Flexibility _____

DAY 2:

Morning _____

Midday _____

Evening _____

Snacks _____

____ Meat	☐ Prayer
____ Bread	☐ Bible Study
____ Vegetable	☐ Scripture Reading
____ Fruit	☐ Memory Verse
____ Milk	☐ Encouragement
____ Fat	____ Water

Exercise
Aerobic _____
Strength _____
Flexibility _____

DAY 3:

Morning _____

Midday _____

Evening _____

Snacks _____

____ Meat	☐ Prayer
____ Bread	☐ Bible Study
____ Vegetable	☐ Scripture Reading
____ Fruit	☐ Memory Verse
____ Milk	☐ Encouragement
____ Fat	____ Water

Exercise
Aerobic _____
Strength _____
Flexibility _____

DAY 4:

Morning _____

Midday _____

Evening _____

Snacks _____

____ Meat	☐ Prayer
____ Bread	☐ Bible Study
____ Vegetable	☐ Scripture Reading
____ Fruit	☐ Memory Verse
____ Milk	☐ Encouragement
____ Fat	____ Water

Exercise
Aerobic _____
Strength _____
Flexibility _____

FIRST PLACE CR

Date _____ through _____
Week # _____ Calorie Level _____

Daily Exchange Plan

Level	Meat	Bread	Veggie	Fruit	Milk	Fat
1200	4-5	5-6	3	2-3	2-3	3-4
1400	5-6	6-7	3-4	3-4	2-3	3-4
1500	5-6	7-8	3-4	3-4	2-3	3-4
1600	6-7	8-9	3-4	3-4	2-3	3-4
1800	6-7	10-11	3-4	3-4	2-3	4-5
2000	6-7	11-12	4-5	4-5	2-3	4-5
2200	7-8	12-13	4-5	4-5	2-3	6-7
2400	8-9	13-14	4-5	4-5	2-3	7-8
2600	9-10	14-15	5	5	2-3	7-8
2800	9-10	15-16	5	5	2-3	9

You may always choose the high range of vegetables and fruits. Limit your high range selections to only one of the following: meat, bread, milk or fat.

Weekly Progress

_____ Loss _____ Gain _____ Maintain

_____ Attendance   _____ Bible Study
_____ Prayer   _____ Scripture Reading
_____ Memory Verse   _____ CR
_____ Encouragement: _____
_____ Exercise
_____ Aerobic
_____ Strength
_____ Flexibility

DAY 5: Date _____

Morning _____

Midday _____

Evening _____

Snacks _____

_____ Meat   ☐ Prayer
_____ Bread   ☐ Bible Study
_____ Vegetable ☐ Scripture Reading
_____ Fruit   ☐ Memory Verse
_____ Milk   ☐ Encouragement
_____ Fat   Water _____

Exercise
Aerobic _____
Strength _____
Flexibility _____

DAY 6: Date _____

Morning _____

Midday _____

Evening _____

Snacks _____

_____ Meat   ☐ Prayer
_____ Bread   ☐ Bible Study
_____ Vegetable ☐ Scripture Reading
_____ Fruit   ☐ Memory Verse
_____ Milk   ☐ Encouragement
_____ Fat   Water _____

Exercise
Aerobic _____
Strength _____
Flexibility _____

DAY 7: Date _____

Morning _____

Midday _____

Evening _____

Snacks _____

_____ Meat   ☐ Prayer
_____ Bread   ☐ Bible Study
_____ Vegetable ☐ Scripture Reading
_____ Fruit   ☐ Memory Verse
_____ Milk   ☐ Encouragement
_____ Fat   Water _____

Exercise
Aerobic _____
Strength _____
Flexibility _____

DAY 1: Date _____

Morning _____

Midday _____

Evening _____

Snacks _____

___ Meat ☐ Prayer
___ Bread ☐ Bible Study
___ Vegetable ☐ Scripture Reading
___ Fruit ☐ Memory Verse
___ Milk ☐ Encouragement
___ Fat ___ Water

Exercise
Aerobic _____
Strength _____
Flexibility _____

DAY 2: Date _____

Morning _____

Midday _____

Evening _____

Snacks _____

___ Meat ☐ Prayer
___ Bread ☐ Bible Study
___ Vegetable ☐ Scripture Reading
___ Fruit ☐ Memory Verse
___ Milk ☐ Encouragement
___ Fat ___ Water

Exercise
Aerobic _____
Strength _____
Flexibility _____

DAY 3: Date _____

Morning _____

Midday _____

Evening _____

Snacks _____

___ Meat ☐ Prayer
___ Bread ☐ Bible Study
___ Vegetable ☐ Scripture Reading
___ Fruit ☐ Memory Verse
___ Milk ☐ Encouragement
___ Fat ___ Water

Exercise
Aerobic _____
Strength _____
Flexibility _____

DAY 4: Date _____

Morning _____

Midday _____

Evening _____

Snacks _____

___ Meat ☐ Prayer
___ Bread ☐ Bible Study
___ Vegetable ☐ Scripture Reading
___ Fruit ☐ Memory Verse
___ Milk ☐ Encouragement
___ Fat ___ Water

Exercise
Aerobic _____
Strength _____
Flexibility _____

FIRST PLACE CR

Name _____

Date _____ through _____

Week # _____ Calorie Level _____

Daily Exchange Plan

Level	Meat	Bread	Veggie	Fruit	Milk	Fat
1200	4-5	5-6	3	2-3	2-3	3-4
1400	5-6	6-7	3-4	3-4	2-3	3-4
1500	5-6	7-8	3-4	3-4	2-3	3-4
1600	6-7	8-9	3-4	3-4	2-3	3-4
1800	6-7	10-11	3-4	3-4	2-3	4-5
2000	6-7	11-12	4-5	4-5	2-3	4-5
2200	7-8	12-13	4-5	4-5	2-3	6-7
2400	8-9	13-14	4-5	4-5	2-3	7-8
2600	9-10	14-15	5	5	2-3	7-8
2800	9-10	15-16	5	5	2-3	9

You may always choose the high range of vegetables and fruits. Limit your high range selections to only one of the following: meat, bread, milk or fat.

Weekly Progress

___ Loss ___ Gain ___ Maintain

___ Attendance ___ Bible Study
___ Prayer ___ Scripture Reading
___ Memory Verse ___ CR
___ Encouragement:
___ Exercise
___ Aerobic

___ Strength
___ Flexibility

DAY 5: Date _____

Morning _____

Midday _____

Evening _____

Snacks _____

___ Meat _____   □ Prayer
___ Bread _____   □ Bible Study
___ Vegetable _____   □ Scripture Reading
___ Fruit _____   □ Memory Verse
___ Milk _____   □ Encouragement
___ Fat _____   Water _____

Exercise
Aerobic _____

Strength _____
Flexibility _____

DAY 6: Date _____

Morning _____

Midday _____

Evening _____

Snacks _____

___ Meat _____   □ Prayer
___ Bread _____   □ Bible Study
___ Vegetable _____   □ Scripture Reading
___ Fruit _____   □ Memory Verse
___ Milk _____   □ Encouragement
___ Fat _____   Water _____

Exercise
Aerobic _____

Strength _____
Flexibility _____

DAY 7: Date _____

Morning _____

Midday _____

Evening _____

Snacks _____

___ Meat _____   □ Prayer
___ Bread _____   □ Bible Study
___ Vegetable _____   □ Scripture Reading
___ Fruit _____   □ Memory Verse
___ Milk _____   □ Encouragement
___ Fat _____   Water _____

Exercise
Aerobic _____

Strength _____
Flexibility _____

DAY 1: Date _____

Morning _____

Midday _____

Evening _____

Snacks _____

___ Meat ___	☐ Prayer	
___ Bread ___	☐ Bible Study	
___ Vegetable ___	☐ Scripture Reading	
___ Fruit ___	☐ Memory Verse	
___ Milk ___	☐ Encouragement	
___ Fat ___ Water ___		

Exercise
Aerobic _____
Strength _____
Flexibility _____

DAY 2: Date _____

Morning _____

Midday _____

Evening _____

Snacks _____

___ Meat ___	☐ Prayer	
___ Bread ___	☐ Bible Study	
___ Vegetable ___	☐ Scripture Reading	
___ Fruit ___	☐ Memory Verse	
___ Milk ___	☐ Encouragement	
___ Fat ___ Water ___		

Exercise
Aerobic _____
Strength _____
Flexibility _____

DAY 3: Date _____

Morning _____

Midday _____

Evening _____

Snacks _____

___ Meat ___	☐ Prayer	
___ Bread ___	☐ Bible Study	
___ Vegetable ___	☐ Scripture Reading	
___ Fruit ___	☐ Memory Verse	
___ Milk ___	☐ Encouragement	
___ Fat ___ Water ___		

Exercise
Aerobic _____
Strength _____
Flexibility _____

DAY 4: Date _____

Morning _____

Midday _____

Evening _____

Snacks _____

___ Meat ___	☐ Prayer	
___ Bread ___	☐ Bible Study	
___ Vegetable ___	☐ Scripture Reading	
___ Fruit ___	☐ Memory Verse	
___ Milk ___	☐ Encouragement	
___ Fat ___ Water ___		

Exercise
Aerobic _____
Strength _____
Flexibility _____

FIRST PLACE CR

Name _____

Date _____ through _____

Week # _____ Calorie Level _____

Daily Exchange Plan

Level	Meat	Bread	Veggie	Fruit	Milk	Fat
1200	4-5	5-6	3	2-3	2-3	3-4
1400	5-6	6-7	3-4	3-4	2-3	3-4
1500	5-6	7-8	3-4	3-4	2-3	3-4
1600	6-7	8-9	3-4	3-4	2-3	3-4
1800	6-7	10-11	3-4	3-4	2-3	4-5
2000	6-7	11-12	4-5	4-5	2-3	4-5
2200	7-8	12-13	4-5	4-5	2-3	6-7
2400	8-9	13-14	4-5	4-5	2-3	7-8
2600	9-10	14-15	5	5	2-3	7-8
2800	9-10	15-16	5	5	2-3	9

You may always choose the high range of vegetables and fruits. Limit your high range selections to only one of the following: meat, bread, milk or fat.

Weekly Progress

_____ Loss _____ Gain _____ Maintain

_____ Attendance _____ Bible Study
_____ Prayer _____ Scripture Reading
_____ Memory Verse _____ CR
_____ Encouragement:
_____ Exercise
_____ Aerobic

Strength _____
Flexibility _____

DAY 7: Date _____

Morning _____

Midday _____

Evening _____

Snacks _____

_____ Meat ☐ Prayer
_____ Bread ☐ Bible Study
_____ Vegetable ☐ Scripture Reading
_____ Fruit ☐ Memory Verse
_____ Milk ☐ Encouragement
_____ Fat Water _____

Exercise
Aerobic _____

Strength _____
Flexibility _____

DAY 6: Date _____

Morning _____

Midday _____

Evening _____

Snacks _____

_____ Meat ☐ Prayer
_____ Bread ☐ Bible Study
_____ Vegetable ☐ Scripture Reading
_____ Fruit ☐ Memory Verse
_____ Milk ☐ Encouragement
_____ Fat Water _____

Exercise
Aerobic _____

Strength _____
Flexibility _____

DAY 5: Date _____

Morning _____

Midday _____

Evening _____

Snacks _____

_____ Meat ☐ Prayer
_____ Bread ☐ Bible Study
_____ Vegetable ☐ Scripture Reading
_____ Fruit ☐ Memory Verse
_____ Milk ☐ Encouragement
_____ Fat Water _____

Exercise
Aerobic _____

Strength _____
Flexibility _____

DAY 1: Date _____ **DAY 2:** Date _____ **DAY 3:** Date _____ **DAY 4:** Date _____

DAY 1

Morning _____

Midday _____

Evening _____

Snacks _____

_____ Meat ☐ Prayer
_____ Bread ☐ Bible Study
_____ Vegetable ☐ Scripture Reading
_____ Fruit ☐ Memory Verse
_____ Milk ☐ Encouragement
_____ Fat _____ Water

Exercise
Aerobic _____
Strength _____
Flexibility _____

DAY 2

Morning _____

Midday _____

Evening _____

Snacks _____

_____ Meat ☐ Prayer
_____ Bread ☐ Bible Study
_____ Vegetable ☐ Scripture Reading
_____ Fruit ☐ Memory Verse
_____ Milk ☐ Encouragement
_____ Fat _____ Water

Exercise
Aerobic _____
Strength _____
Flexibility _____

DAY 3

Morning _____

Midday _____

Evening _____

Snacks _____

_____ Meat ☐ Prayer
_____ Bread ☐ Bible Study
_____ Vegetable ☐ Scripture Reading
_____ Fruit ☐ Memory Verse
_____ Milk ☐ Encouragement
_____ Fat _____ Water

Exercise
Aerobic _____
Strength _____
Flexibility _____

DAY 4

Morning _____

Midday _____

Evening _____

Snacks _____

_____ Meat ☐ Prayer
_____ Bread ☐ Bible Study
_____ Vegetable ☐ Scripture Reading
_____ Fruit ☐ Memory Verse
_____ Milk ☐ Encouragement
_____ Fat _____ Water

Exercise
Aerobic _____
Strength _____
Flexibility _____

FIRST PLACE CR

Name _____

Date _____ through _____

Week # _____ Calorie Level _____

Daily Exchange Plan

Level	Meat	Bread	Veggie	Fruit	Milk	Fat
1200	4-5	5-6	3	2-3	2-3	3-4
1400	5-6	6-7	3-4	3-4	2-3	3-4
1500	5-6	7-8	3-4	3-4	2-3	3-4
1600	6-7	8-9	3-4	3-4	2-3	3-4
1800	6-7	10-11	3-4	3-4	2-3	4-5
2000	6-7	11-12	4-5	4-5	2-3	4-5
2200	7-8	12-13	4-5	4-5	2-3	6-7
2400	8-9	13-14	4-5	4-5	2-3	7-8
2600	9-10	14-15	5	5	2-3	7-8
2800	9-10	15-16	5	5	2-3	9

You may always choose the high range of vegetables and fruits. Limit your high range selections to only one of the following: meat, bread, milk or fat.

Weekly Progress

_____ Loss _____ Gain _____ Maintain

_____ Attendance _____ Bible Study
_____ Prayer _____ Scripture Reading
_____ Memory Verse _____ CR
_____ Encouragement:
_____ Exercise
Aerobic _____

Strength _____
Flexibility _____

DAY 5: Date _____

Morning _____
_____

Midday _____
_____

Evening _____
_____

Snacks _____
_____

_____ Meat   ☐ Prayer
_____ Bread   ☐ Bible Study
_____ Vegetable ☐ Scripture Reading
_____ Fruit   ☐ Memory Verse
_____ Milk   ☐ Encouragement
_____ Fat   Water _____

Exercise
Aerobic _____

Strength _____
Flexibility _____

DAY 6: Date _____

Morning _____
_____

Midday _____
_____

Evening _____
_____

Snacks _____
_____

_____ Meat   ☐ Prayer
_____ Bread   ☐ Bible Study
_____ Vegetable ☐ Scripture Reading
_____ Fruit   ☐ Memory Verse
_____ Milk   ☐ Encouragement
_____ Fat   Water _____

Exercise
Aerobic _____

Strength _____
Flexibility _____

DAY 7: Date _____

Morning _____
_____

Midday _____
_____

Evening _____
_____

Snacks _____
_____

_____ Meat   ☐ Prayer
_____ Bread   ☐ Bible Study
_____ Vegetable ☐ Scripture Reading
_____ Fruit   ☐ Memory Verse
_____ Milk   ☐ Encouragement
_____ Fat   Water _____

Exercise
Aerobic _____

Strength _____
Flexibility _____

DAY 1: Date _____

Morning _____

Midday _____

Evening _____

Snacks _____

___ Meat	☐ Prayer
___ Bread	☐ Bible Study
___ Vegetable	☐ Scripture Reading
___ Fruit	☐ Memory Verse
___ Milk	☐ Encouragement
___ Fat	___ Water

Exercise
Aerobic _____
Strength _____
Flexibility _____

DAY 2: Date _____

Morning _____

Midday _____

Evening _____

Snacks _____

___ Meat	☐ Prayer
___ Bread	☐ Bible Study
___ Vegetable	☐ Scripture Reading
___ Fruit	☐ Memory Verse
___ Milk	☐ Encouragement
___ Fat	___ Water

Exercise
Aerobic _____
Strength _____
Flexibility _____

DAY 3: Date _____

Morning _____

Midday _____

Evening _____

Snacks _____

___ Meat	☐ Prayer
___ Bread	☐ Bible Study
___ Vegetable	☐ Scripture Reading
___ Fruit	☐ Memory Verse
___ Milk	☐ Encouragement
___ Fat	___ Water

Exercise
Aerobic _____
Strength _____
Flexibility _____

DAY 4: Date _____

Morning _____

Midday _____

Evening _____

Snacks _____

___ Meat	☐ Prayer
___ Bread	☐ Bible Study
___ Vegetable	☐ Scripture Reading
___ Fruit	☐ Memory Verse
___ Milk	☐ Encouragement
___ Fat	___ Water

Exercise
Aerobic _____
Strength _____
Flexibility _____

FIRST PLACE CR

Name _____

Date _____ through _____

Week # _____ Calorie Level _____

Daily Exchange Plan

Level	Meat	Bread	Veggie	Fruit	Milk	Fat
1200	4-5	5-6	3	2-3	2-3	3-4
1400	5-6	6-7	3-4	3-4	2-3	3-4
1500	5-6	7-8	3-4	3-4	2-3	3-4
1600	6-7	8-9	3-4	3-4	2-3	3-4
1800	6-7	10-11	3-4	3-4	2-3	4-5
2000	6-7	11-12	4-5	4-5	2-3	4-5
2200	7-8	12-13	4-5	4-5	2-3	6-7
2400	8-9	13-14	4-5	4-5	2-3	7-8
2600	9-10	14-15	5	5	2-3	7-8
2800	9-10	15-16	5	5	2-3	9

You may always choose the high range of vegetables and fruits. Limit your high range selections to only one of the following: meat, bread, milk or fat.

Weekly Progress

_____ Loss _____ Gain _____ Maintain

_____ Attendance _____ Bible Study

_____ Prayer _____ Scripture Reading

_____ Memory Verse _____ CR

_____ Encouragement:

_____ Exercise

Aerobic _____

Strength _____

Flexibility _____

DAY 5: Date _____

Morning _____

Midday _____

Evening _____

Snacks _____

_____ Meat   ☐ Prayer
_____ Bread   ☐ Bible Study
_____ Vegetable   ☐ Scripture Reading
_____ Fruit   ☐ Memory Verse
_____ Milk   ☐ Encouragement
_____ Fat   _____ Water

Exercise
Aerobic _____

Strength _____
Flexibility _____

DAY 6: Date _____

Morning _____

Midday _____

Evening _____

Snacks _____

_____ Meat   ☐ Prayer
_____ Bread   ☐ Bible Study
_____ Vegetable   ☐ Scripture Reading
_____ Fruit   ☐ Memory Verse
_____ Milk   ☐ Encouragement
_____ Fat   _____ Water

Exercise
Aerobic _____

Strength _____
Flexibility _____

DAY 7: Date _____

Morning _____

Midday _____

Evening _____

Snacks _____

_____ Meat   ☐ Prayer
_____ Bread   ☐ Bible Study
_____ Vegetable   ☐ Scripture Reading
_____ Fruit   ☐ Memory Verse
_____ Milk   ☐ Encouragement
_____ Fat   _____ Water

Exercise
Aerobic _____

Strength _____
Flexibility _____

DAY 1: Date _____

Morning _____

Midday _____

Evening _____

Snacks _____

- ☐ Prayer
- ☐ Bible Study
- ☐ Scripture Reading
- ☐ Memory Verse
- ☐ Encouragement

Meat _____
Bread _____
Vegetable _____
Fruit _____
Milk _____
Fat _____
Water _____

Exercise
Aerobic _____
Strength _____
Flexibility _____

DAY 2: Date _____

Morning _____

Midday _____

Evening _____

Snacks _____

- ☐ Prayer
- ☐ Bible Study
- ☐ Scripture Reading
- ☐ Memory Verse
- ☐ Encouragement

Meat _____
Bread _____
Vegetable _____
Fruit _____
Milk _____
Fat _____
Water _____

Exercise
Aerobic _____
Strength _____
Flexibility _____

DAY 3: Date _____

Morning _____

Midday _____

Evening _____

Snacks _____

- ☐ Prayer
- ☐ Bible Study
- ☐ Scripture Reading
- ☐ Memory Verse
- ☐ Encouragement

Meat _____
Bread _____
Vegetable _____
Fruit _____
Milk _____
Fat _____
Water _____

Exercise
Aerobic _____
Strength _____
Flexibility _____

DAY 4: Date _____

Morning _____

Midday _____

Evening _____

Snacks _____

- ☐ Prayer
- ☐ Bible Study
- ☐ Scripture Reading
- ☐ Memory Verse
- ☐ Encouragement

Meat _____
Bread _____
Vegetable _____
Fruit _____
Milk _____
Fat _____
Water _____

Exercise
Aerobic _____
Strength _____
Flexibility _____

CONTRIBUTORS

Jody Wilkinson, M.D., M.S., the writer of the Wellness Worksheets for this study, is a physician and exercise physiologist at the Cooper Institute in Dallas, Texas. He trained at the University of Texas Health Science Center in San Antonio, Texas, and Baylor University Medical Center in Dallas. Dr. Wilkinson conducts research on physical activity, nutrition and weight management and has worked with the American Heart Association to develop a health program. He believes strongly in using biblical teaching to motivate people to take care of their physical bodies and enjoy abundant living. Jody and his wife, Natalie, have been married 10 years and have two daughters, Jordan and Sarah, and twin sons, Joel and Cooper.

Scott Wilson, C.E.C., A.A.C., the author of the menu plans in this study, has been cooking professionally for 23 years. A certified executive chef with the American Culinary Federation, he currently works in the Greater Atlanta area as a personal chef and food consultant. Along with serving as the national food consultant for First Place, he is a part-time nutrition teacher at Life University and chef/host of a cable cooking show in the Atlanta area, "Cooking 4 Life." Scott has also authored two cookbooks, *Dining Under the Magnolia* and *Healthy Home Cooking*. In his spare time, he is active in church work and spends time with his wife of 18 years, Jennifer, and their daughter, Katie.

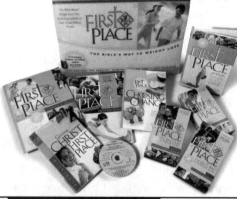